CORPORATE
BITCH TO
SHAMAN

EVELYN M. BRODIE

CORPORATE BITCH TO SHAMAN

A journey uncovering the links between
21st century science,
consciousness
and the ancient healing practices

Matador
9 Priory Business Park
Kibworth Beauchamp
Leicestershire LE8 0RX, UK
Tel: (+44) 116 279 2299
Fax: (+44) 116 279 2277
Email: books@troubador.co.uk
Web: www.troubador.co.uk/matador

ISBN 978 1783060 627

British Library Cataloguing in Publication Data.
A catalogue record for this book is available from the British Library.

Typeset in StempelGaramond Roman by Troubador Publishing Ltd
Printed and bound in the UK by TJ International, Padstow, Cornwall
Illustrations by Carita Keranen
Cover Photograph by George Christie

Matador is an imprint of Troubador Publishing Ltd

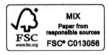

This book is dedicated to all my teachers:
My parents
My children
My lovers
My biological lineage
My karmic lineage
My gurus
My friends
And my clients – each and every one of whom brings their own life experience and teaches me something new

Contents

Acknowledgements

I give deep thanks to the friends and professional experts in various fields who read part or all of the early versions of this work and contributed such valuable comments, especially Deike Begg, Dr. Harry Bush, George Christie, Hye Yoon Chung, Katrina Ferron, Joel Feyerherm, Carita Keranen, Andrew Klein, Sandy Munro, Dr. Govin Murugachandran, Hannah Northern, Lord O'Donnell, Joanne Perez, Dr. Locksley Ryan, 'Sean' and Lindsay Williams.

I owe huge gratitude to Jasmin Naim for proofreading early versions of the manuscript and for encouragement and information about the publishing process. Ben Belenus and Gemma Wilson were also generous with their time and support regarding the publishing process.

Particular gratitude goes to my best friend George, who supported me, encouraged me and believed in me as this project developed. Thanks also to all those at Matador Publishing who have been of such assistance in turning my manuscript into reality.

I also gratefully acknowledge the following authors and publishers for giving me permission to reprint quotations from their publications.

Begg, Deike. 1999. Rebirthing, *Freedom From Your Past.* HarperCollins Publishers Ltd.

Bohm, David. 1980. *Wholeness and the Implicate Order.* Routledge & Paul Kegan/Taylor & Francis Books (UK)

Candace B. Pert. 1997. *Molecules of Emotion.* RAPID Pharmaceuticals, AG, Maryland, USA and Scribner Publishing Group

Church, Dawson. 2007. *The Genie in Your Genes.* Elite Books

Piero Ferrucci. 1982. *What We May Be.* Piero Ferrucci (UK) and Penguin Group (USA) Inc.

Hawking, Stephen and Mlodinow, Leonard. 2010.*The Grand Design.* Bantam Press, The Random House Group, Bantam Press

Lipton, Bruce. 2005.*The Biology of Belief.* Hay House, Inc., Carlsbad, CA

Narby, Jeremy. 1999. *The Cosmic Serpent.* Penguin Group (USA rights) Inc,/ Barbara Moulton, The Moulton Agency, California (UK rights)

Osho. 2000. *New Man for the New Millennium.* Osho International Foundation, www.osho.com/copyrights

Schlitz, Marilyn, Amorok, Tina with Micozzi, Marc S.. 2005. *Consciousness and Healing.* Elsevier

Singh Khalsa, M.D., Dharma and Stauth, Cameron. 2001. *Meditation as Medicine.: Activate the Power of Your Natural Healing Force.* Gallery Publishing Group

Sri Aurobindo, 1952. *The Problem of Rebirth.* Sri Aurobindo Ashram Trust

Targ, Russell. 2004. *Limitless Mind.* New World Library, www.NewWorldLibrary.com

Villoldo, Alberto. 2005. *Mending the Past and Healing the Future with Soul Retrieval.* Hay House, Inc., Carlsbad, CA

Finally I would like to thank The Monroe Institute for allowing me to quote extracts of their research from their website http://www.monroeinstitute.org/research/overview-of-research-at-the-monroe-institute

Any errors and omissions are of course my own.

I would love to hear from any of you who read this book, especially about the areas where there may be more recent research that I am unaware of. Please contact me through balanceandpurposehealing@gmail.com

My healing website with full information about the services and workshops that I offer is at www.balanceandpurpose.co.uk

Introduction

This is my story, my journey over the six years 2004 to 2010, during which time I did a u-turn from working in a succession of demanding, stressful jobs, where I had embraced the role of 'corporate bitch' to living and working as a shaman and energy healer. My personal story is interwoven with the scientific and medical knowledge that I discovered as I struggled to rationally validate the experiences I was having.

Much of what I have discovered along the way I would have labelled as ridiculous nonsense a decade ago. But if we don't ask the right questions we don't get the right answers! And a decade ago I was definitely not asking the kinds of questions I focus on today.

On my journey I have attended many amazing courses and have worked with a wide variety of teachers and therapists, from many different cultures and belief systems. I have travelled to North America, Central America, South America, India, Thailand and Laos, studying and working with shamans from different tribes, Buddhists, Hindus, Tantrikas, psychotherapists from different schools and a huge variety of energy healers.

I am not a physicist, a biologist, a yogi or a psychologist. The scientific, medical and mystical research that I have pulled together here is taken from many academic sources across many disciplines. I make no apology for this. There is too much information on this planet for any one person to investigate or become expert in more than a fraction of it first-hand. I have tried to use some of the gifts of being a corporate bitch, including my journalistic techniques, enquiring mind and tenacity, to put together various pieces of the jigsaw into a coherent whole. However I have credited all the primary sources that I've gained my knowledge from and encourage the interested reader to follow up in these varied fields.

The scientific and medical knowledge presented here is available to those that know where to look, but it is not widely taught. Much of it remains in academia. That is partly because some of it is difficult intellectually and challenging to the way we perceive the world works. It is partly because the latest findings on the links between our widely defined 'environment' (including our family, what we eat, the toxins we inhale, the lifestyle we choose and what we think) and our health, give us far more choice over our health than the medical establishment and the pharmaceutical companies would have us believe.

I believe this knowledge needs to be much more widely disseminated, becoming embedded into our educational system, our media and our healthcare system to allow each one of us to step into our full potential as co-creators of our lives and our health, rather than being victims of our conditioning and circumstances.

So, I invite you to join me as I describe my journey from corporate bitch to shaman. I hope you will be sufficiently intrigued and challenged as you follow my journey and my discoveries of how 21st century science is evolving to validate the ancient healing wisdoms of the indigenous peoples around the world, to continue with additional research and reading from the sources I provide. I would be delighted if my story encourages you to progress on your own path of self-development and to explore the wide range of altered states of consciousness that I have discovered allow connection with the universal energy field.

London, April 2013

Chapter 1:

Beginnings

'We see what we believe, and not just the contrary; and to change what we see, it is sometimes necessary to change what we believe.'[1] (Jeremy Narby)

If you had suggested to me a decade ago that today I would be a shaman[2], an energy healer, holistic body-worker, Reiki Master, craniosacral therapist and tantrika, I would have said you were nuts, delusional, lunatic! This book is the story of how my experiences over the last eight years have led me to change my belief system and adopt a new way of living.

I spent thirty years competing largely against men in the driven, rational, intellectual worlds of government, the City, journalism and strategic communications advice to the uber-rich. For many years I stepped into the role of 'corporate bitch', largely suppressing my femininity, sexuality, intuition and compassion, without even being aware of the harsh image I was projecting to the world.

Friends who have known me for more than thirty years now admit I used to be scary and formidable, although they wouldn't

---

[1] Narby, Jeremy. 1999. *The Cosmic Serpent, DNA and the Origins of Knowledge.* p.140 New York, NY, USA: Jeremy P. Tarcher/Putnam
[2] My definition of a shaman is a healer working with causes rather than symptoms, often in the energy field. Someone capable of altering their state of consciousness to work outside linear space and time.

have dared say that to the corporate bitch! I was definitely driven by my left-brain, logical, uncompromising, judgemental, intolerant and selfish. I didn't really care about the problems of the world. I didn't do any sort of charitable work or even giving. My focus was entirely on the well-being and consumption of myself and my family.

My husband and I appeared to the outside world to have it all. We were affluent, with high-powered jobs, a boy, a girl, a nanny, a fun convertible car and a kiddie car. We spent a ridiculous amount of money on fine wining and dining in some of the best restaurants in London and amazing holidays at beautiful chateaux, chalets and resorts throughout Europe and North America. This was the 1980s in London, so of course we also had the requisite Victorian house and scoured the antique fairs and markets for suitable 'period' furniture and objets d'art.

Right from the start I would like to make it clear that I did **not** have any religious or spiritual beliefs before I had the experiences described in this book. I was brought up in a strict Scottish Protestant family where morality seemed to consist of doing things because they were 'right' and if you didn't do them, or broke the mould, you would suffer in hell for eternity. So there was no sense of joy, compassion, or empathy, and certainly no expression of emotions. Just hard work, obligation, repression. It seemed to me as if I was being taught that God had determined that everything joyful was sinful.

By age seven or eight I rejected this view of God and with it ditched all forms of organised religion (including refusing to go to Sunday School), much to the dismay of my parents. My father was particularly distressed. He had been brought up in a very poor, war-torn Glasgow and for him hard work and material success, discipline and self-denial were paramount. However, although I mentally rejected this view of God and Christianity, for many years I never did quite manage to escape my Protestant conditioning about the necessity for a strong work ethic and a sexual 'morality'. I held on to a belief that success was measured in financial terms and that for a woman in particular to enjoy sex was wrong – it was dirty and sinful. Nice girls didn't do it, and when they had to, within the confines of marriage, they certainly didn't enjoy it!

The result of this conditioning was that for thirty years of my life I worked and played hard, achieved excellent academic credentials and had a varied, interesting, and successful career. I started out as a professional economist with the Government in the Treasury and Cabinet Office and then in the City with an investment bank. Whilst there I became a frequent guest on financial television and radio shows, discussing interest rates, exchange rates, growth, inflation, house prices, investment opportunities and so on. It was the eighties so I came complete with curly perm, designer suits, shoulder pads and stilettos. My greatest claim to fame was predicting the housing collapse of the early 1990s, which seemed inevitable after the Chancellor of the Exchequer at the time, Nigel Lawson, announced the removal of multiple tax relief on mortgage interest, in April 1988, to be replaced by a single relief per property to take effect in August. This led to a final stampede into the housing market, inflating what was already a substantial bubble.

This prediction gave me a lot of radio and television air-time, talking about the property market and I developed good connections with financial TV programmes. After my son was born (the first of my two children) I decided I could no longer travel around the world talking to investors and fund managers. The bank I had been working for co-incidentally got taken over at around the same time and my share options became valuable, so I cashed them in and moved from the City to the BBC where I became a financial journalist. I continued as an on-air economics and financial commentator for thirteen years, working in a variety of broadcasting environments, including Sky Business, CNBC and Bloomberg.

I then left journalism to become head of corporate and financial communication at a FTSE 100 company, before finishing my corporate career as a consultant with a strategic communications company dealing with a variety of clients from charities and non-government organisations, to super rich Russian and Eastern European oligarchs.

Despite the outward success, for the first forty-five years of my life, whilst working in that corporate environment and being driven by financial measures of happiness and success, I also felt very judged. I was obsessed by what people thought about me!

I appeared confident and controlling, but that was my mask. I had very little self-esteem and depended on the approval of others, particularly men, both in my personal life and the workplace.

Throughout that time I firmly believed that when I die my body will be cremated and that will be the end of me. Dust to dust, ashes to ashes. I hoped I'd be remembered by my friends and children for as long as they lived, for the happy times we had spent together, but I knew I wouldn't have contributed anything of lasting historic importance or significance. I accepted that only a few become famous or infamous enough to be immortalised and I didn't consider myself to be amongst that chosen few. I thought I was happy in my belief that once the physical body is dead, there is nothing else beyond that, so we should enjoy it while we can.

The journey I have been on in recent years came as a complete shock to me! It wasn't something I had always wanted to do. My long term dream until 2004 was to accumulate enough money to buy a vineyard and villa in Tuscany for an early retirement, eating fine Italian food and quaffing Chianti.

But somehow, after stumbling on a few pages in a book that piqued my attention in 2002, I got hooked into a path of enquiry that has opened doors I didn't even know existed.

The initial experience which changed my life came in November 2004, at a beautiful retreat centre in Wales. This epiphany is described in detail in the next chapter, but it forced me to change my belief system. After that first exposure to an alternative state of consciousness I began an intense period of investigation and learning. This has included:

- A series of 'rebirthing' sessions (described in Chapter 4)
- Attending two 'out of body' courses at the Monroe Institute in Virginia, USA (described in Chapters 5 and 6)
- Completing the Foundation course in Psychosynthesis transpersonal psychotherapy
- Training as a Reiki Master
- Completing the two year training in craniosacral therapy at the London College of Craniosacral Therapy
- Completing Dr. Alberto Villoldo's shamanic Medicine

Wheel training in Germany, Holland and the UK (described in Chapter 11)
- Working with Roger Woolger and his colleagues on past life regression techniques
- Hiking the Sacred Valley in Peru with Jose Luis Herrara of the Rainbow Jaguar Institute, based in Cusco and a selection of Peruvian shamans
- Working with Don Alfredo, a Shipibo shaman, and the plant medicine in the Peruvian Amazon (described in Chapter 12)
- Participating in two ten-day long tantric courses led by Ma Ananda Sarita at Osho Nisarga in Northern India.

During most of this time I was still working in the corporate sector. Apart from anything else I needed the money, as these courses and trips were expensive. I was also constantly working with a succession of personal therapists and in my spare time, apart from looking after two teenage children, I was pounding through books on quantum physics, psychoneuroimmunology[3], epigenetics[4] and meditation.

It was an intense and exhausting period when I slept very little. I seemed to need thirty hours in every day and my children fended for themselves a lot, inducing a guilt which I have tried to atone for more recently. It was a conflicted time, with different aspects of myself pulling me in very different directions. As I progressed to my new path a number of my old acquaintances and colleagues dropped away, as they could not accept the new direction I was taking. I know now that my true friends of course have supported me throughout the journey and a number of them are named in the acknowledgments. Like love, true friendship is non-judgemental and unconditional!

---

[3] Psychoneuroimmunology is the area of medical research which connects our thoughts (psyche), our nervous system (neurology) and our immune system to prove that what we think affects our health.
[4] Epigenetics is the science of how environmental signals select, modify and regulate gene activity leading to heritable changes in gene function that occur without a change in the DNA sequence.

Finally, in June 2010, with my children reaching adulthood and independence, I felt ready to step fully into my new life as a shaman, energy healer and body-worker. I quit the consultancy I was working at and left for a seven month trip. That time was a combination of learning and relaxing. I spent a month in Peru working with shamans before heading for four months of meditation, tantra and sight-seeing in India, then a month each in Thailand and Laos. In January 2011 I returned to London to work full time in my new profession of shaman and energy healer.

Many of the personal experiences I describe in this book involve altered states of consciousness, induced by a variety of methods. These altered states of consciousness allow us to access images drawn from our personal history, from nature, from the collective unconscious and even from the cosmos. In particular they allow us to access information from a different place and time from where our physical bodies are located.

If you have never experimented with such altered states of consciousness, please don't put the book down at this point as 'New Age gobbledy-gook'. I would have found the statement I have made above really difficult to accept just a few years ago, and I know that it is only by **experiencing for oneself** the potential that we all have to exist outside the physical body, that one can know it to be true.

Stanislav Grof has been at the forefront of the scientific investigation of altered states of consciousness and transpersonal experiences for over forty-five years, principally accessed using particular patterns and methods of breathing known as holotropic breathwork[5]. He writes, *'Researchers who have studied and/or personally experienced these fascinating phenomena realize that the attempts of mainstream science to dismiss them as irrelevant products of human fantasy and imagination or as hallucinations – erratic products of pathological processes in the brain – are naive and inadequate. Any unbiased study of the transpersonal domain*

---

[5] Holotropic breathwork was evolved by Stanislav Grof as a way of accessing altered states of consciousness. It derives from the Greek holos, meaning 'whole' and trepein, meaning 'to turn or direct towards a thing'.

of the psyche has to come to the conclusion that the observations represent a critical challenge not only for psychiatry and psychology but for the entire philosophy of Western science.'[6]

One of the purposes of this book is to open the doors that I stumbled upon to others, as I believe that what lies behind them is incredibly important and should be knowledge available to everyone, to allow people to take better control of their lives and make more informed decisions.

Some of the experiences that I describe as I tell the story of this transformational journey were initially frightening, as they involved either a loss of control by my rational mind or a descent into difficult, repressed areas deep within my unconscious mind. The first rebirthing, many of the shamanic exercises, transpersonal psychotherapy and the hallucinations induced by the Amazonian plant medicine ayahuasca all fall into this category.

One of the friends who read an early version of this manuscript asked me afterwards what drove me to continue with my explorations given the apparently scary nature of many of my experiences? Why do I keep opening these new doors, not knowing what is behind them, when it might seem safer and easier to leave them locked shut?

I reflected on those questions and feel there are several answers.

First, I know from both my own experience, conversations with friends who are also on a path of deep self-exploration and healing and work I have done with clients, that we often get the greatest insights from difficult events. Although it may be painful initially to go into what is known in psychotherapy and shamanism as the 'shadow-work', the unpleasant events and traumas that we have repressed (or mistakes we feel we have made), what actually happens is that they make us sick when we leave them to fester. Shit happens in life. If we repress that shit it is still there, eating away in our unconscious mind and impacting the cells of our physical body. The aim of the shadow-work is to acknowledge

---

[6] Grof, Stanislav. 2005. Psychology of the Future: Lessons from Modern Consciousness Research pp 261-262 in *Consciousness and Healing*, edited by Schlitz, Marilyn and Amorok, Tina with Micozzi, Marc S. St Louis, Missouri, USA: Elsevier

those traumas and mistakes, see if there were any gifts or lessons, and then integrate the benefits whilst releasing the suffering from the energy field and the physical body.

Second, I felt incredibly honoured from very early on in my journey of self-discovery to have gained access to some of the teachers and information I was receiving. I knew I could very easily have lived my life without stumbling across the initial books and teachers that changed my own life. So I felt an overwhelming obligation to share the information and teachings I was being given. Somehow I knew I wasn't being given these gifts just for my own selfish use – I was being given them so that I could use the intellectual tools and gifts of my 'corporate bitch' life to reach others with information that they otherwise might not stumble upon.

Third, as a child, I always drove my parents and family crazy. They gave me the nick-name 'How', as I was forever asking how things worked, how things happened? Maybe it is that deep quest for knowledge and wisdom, which made me an irritating child, then a curious, questioning journalist, that has also been a force driving me to self-enquiry, self-improvement and then the answers to the questions that have troubled humanity for centuries.

Along the way I have come to know that many of my previously held beliefs were wrong. Experience has shown me that I am an energy, a soul or spirit, that will exist as a vibration in this or another universe for all time. I also have come to learn that my purpose in this physical body, during this lifetime, is to grow and evolve as much as possible and above all to cultivate love and compassion. For what I do and learn here and now, the karma[7] that I create, will influence the energy that goes on to the next life, and the next, and the next. Those 'lives' may be here on earth, as reincarnations in human form, or they may be elsewhere in space and time as a different type of 'being'. My true essence, which is beyond the physical, is infinite and ever-lasting.

Ten years ago the corporate bitch would have dismissed this statement that I am making today as fucking bollocks. This book is my attempt to present the experiences that initially changed

---

[7] Karma refers to the totality of our actions and their accompanying reactions in this, previous and future lives.

my mind, as well as the scientific and medical evidence that I have discovered is accumulating to support my new views.

Some of this information is without doubt intellectually challenging, which is why it is not more widely publicised. Other portions of it challenge some of the richest, most powerful corporations and institutions on the planet, which I believe is one of the main reasons why those parts are not more widely publicised. I understand why that knowledge is suppressed – I use to work for a number of those powerful institutions!

My hope is that the strength of the accumulated scientific proof and evidence that I present here and my rational, logical, business background will create enough interest and curiosity in those of you who totally deny or denigrate the philosophies of 'New Age hippies', 'psychics', 'energy healers', 'mystics' and so on, to lead you to testing out for yourself one or more of the alternative therapies and philosophies I describe. Only your own direct experience that you are more than your physical body and hence can experience realities beyond your physical boundary will ever persuade you. I know that. No amount of theory, or reading or hearing of the experiences of others can ever substitute for direct experience. That is what changes a hypothesis into a belief and then a known.

Even if you don't want to go down the path of experience, I hope that the scientific and medical knowledge that I present will lead you to a greater curiosity about the uncertain, interconnected world we live in. At various times in the past scientists have believed they were close to an integrated, complete 'theory of everything'. Only in recent years have we begun to realise how little we truly know!

Today, as never before, science is able to provide experimental evidence of the 'non-local' effects that have in the past been assigned (in the Western world at least) to the realm of the paranormal. Over the last thirty years, physicists, biologists and doctors have been accumulating mountains of evidence about non-locality which appears to require either that information can travel faster than the speed of light, or that every particle of the universe is interconnected in some way so that each part instantaneously knows what is happening elsewhere.

Although this evidence about non-locality now exists, widely accepted explanations for it are still lacking. We still don't quite know how it works, although we know it does happen. Chapter 3 sets out in some detail one of the leading theories put forward by David Bohm, one of the best known physicists of the 20th century who attempted to span the worlds of theoretical physics, philosophy and metaphysics, as well as providing sources for a couple of the alternative theories put forward by other scientists.

I believe it is crucial that this knowledge about non-locality reaches everyone. We may not understand it, but we need to know that it is there and that it can influence our lives. Think of all the other things we as individuals don't understand if they are not in our area of expertise. For me that includes how I can talk to someone on the other side of the world using a mobile phone, how airplanes actually stay in the sky and how my laptop works. But we use these technologies all the time. If we at least know of the existence of non-locality and the relatively recent medical discoveries of epigenetics and psychoneuroimmunology, we can use them too. However it is impossible to use them effectively if we don't even know they exist!

The implications of a wider knowledge of and acceptance of this universal phenomenon of non-locality within society at large are enormous. If we recognise that we can access the subconscious, unconscious and collective consciousness, then we can become co-creators of our own health and destiny to a much greater extent than we are frequently led to believe by our parents, our schools, our governments, our doctors and Western society in general.

For many people self-responsibility may be a frightening concept. It is often much easier to choose to be a victim, as that removes our own responsibility for how our life has turned out. Stepping into the role of being co-creators requires us to admit that we are where we are, doing whatever we are doing, because that's where we've chosen to be. We also have choice about the attitude with which we view events and people around us. We can't blame anyone else – the system or our genes or our parents. Each of us has a choice at each moment of each day, on what to do and what to think.

Of course if every individual were to step into a role of greater self-responsibility and empowerment, there would be losers: all the companies and institutions which try to control and manipulate us for whatever ends – usually power or money – would see their influence fade.

Today, helping others achieve their magnificence and potential as co-creators of their own destiny, or at least helping them to wake up in the morning with a sense of hope that their lives can change and have meaning and purpose and that they have choice, is one of my life's purposes. My work with clients is often deep and intense, not over years of therapy, but in just a few sessions. I feel honoured to be allowed to help my clients in this way and I give thanks to them for sharing their stories and allowing me into their energy systems at such a profound level of trust and intimacy.

I can only ask that you read this book bearing in mind this next quote from Stanslav Grof. *'When confronted with the challenging observations from modern consciousness research, we have only two choices. The first one is to reject the new observations simply because they are incompatible with the traditional scientific belief system. This involves an arrogant assumption that we already know what the universe is like and can tell with certainty what is possible and what is not possible... In this context, anyone who brings critically challenging data is accused of being a bad scientist, a fraud, or a mentally deranged person.*

'The second reaction to challenging new observations is characteristic of true science. It is excitement about and intense interest in such anomalies, combined with healthy scepticism... It is hard to imagine that Western science will continue indefinitely to censor all the extraordinary evidence that has in the past been accumulated in the study of various forms of holotropic states, as well as to ignore the influx of new data. Sooner or later, it will have to face this challenge and accept all the far-reaching theoretical and practical consequences. When that happens, we will realize that the nature of human beings is very different from what is being taught at Western universities and what the industrial civilization believes it to be.' [8]

---

[8] Grof, Stanislav. 2005. Psychology of the Future: Lessons from Modern Consciousness Research pp265-66 in *Consciousness and Healing*, edited by Schlitz, Marilyn and Amorok, Tina with Micozzi, Marc S. St Louis, Missouri, USA: Elsevier

Timeline of my journey

Date	Event	Teaching
June 1979	Graduated from Glasgow University, Scotland	1st class Honours in Economics, enabling me to get a job as an economist in H.M. Treasury and then the Cabinet Office
June 1983	Graduated from Stanford University, California	Post-graduate Masters degree in Economics
November 2004	David Morehouse Remote Viewing course	We are more than our physical bodies – something is capable of viewing events distant in space and time.
April 2005	Rebirthing	Going out of body for a prolonged period of time.
May 2005	Sean became my partner	Start of sexual awakening and letting go of guilt and shame.
August 2005	Reiki Level 1 attunement	Starting to use energy healing.
April 2006	Gateway programme at the Monroe Institute	The ability to receive messages from 'guides' or the inforealm.
January – December 2007	Foundation course in Psychosynthesis	Gave me basic counselling skills and on a personal level a year of deep introspection, shadow work and psychotherapy.

January 2007	Lifeline programme at the Monroe Institute	Visiting a past life and re-writing a limiting soul contract. Healing the lineage.
October 2007 – June 2009	Craniosacral Therapy Training	Teachings in anatomy and physiology and the skills to work as a craniosacral therapist.
November 2007	First module of The Medicine Wheel	Further healing of the lineage and knowing that it is 'OK to be a witch'.
August 2008	Working with Jose Luis Herrara in Peru	Learning about the Cosmology and ceremonies of the shamans of the Andes.
November 2009	Introduction to tantra	New understanding of my sexuality and move towards self love.
July 2010	Working with the plant medicine shaman in the Amazon	The cleansing and healing power of the master plants and the way our DNA can access plant knowledge.
January – May 2012	Deep Memory Process course	Techniques for past life regression work with clients and further investigation of my own past lives.

Chapter 2:
Remote Viewing - Opening Pandora's Box

'I have spent over eighteen years of my life striving to be validated, trying to have my efforts accepted by culture. In other words I've subjected myself to thousands of laboratory-approved, controlled, and accepted research protocols. Now, after thousands of judgements and rehashes, with evaluation heaped upon evaluation, I feel I have the right to say that I've been declared a remote viewer of some worth: dependable, able to replicate within the confines of an approved protocol, sometimes sufficiently accurate, and (most importantly) not crazy.[9] (Joseph McMoneagle)

When people ask me what the epiphany was that turned my path around, the answer is Remote Viewing. Although it is not a practice I continue with today, it was the experience that forced me to change my belief system and led me to the man who was to become a teacher (and lover) for the next two years, leading me to books and therapies that I didn't even know existed.

---

[9] McMoneagle, Joseph. 1993. *Mind Trek, Exploring Consciousness, Time and Space Through Remote Viewing*. p.18. Charlottesville, VA, USA: Hampton Roads

The initial catalyst was a reference to the American 'Psychic Spying' or 'Remote Viewing' (RV) programme that started at the Stanford Research Institute, (SRI) California, in 1973. Many people have only heard of RV because of the Hollywood movie *The Men Who Stare at Goats*, which poked fun at the whole RV concept, but the programme was conceived within and funded by the US Department of Defence and staffed largely by highly decorated military officers from 1975 until 1995. Over time it was known in the intelligence community as Scangate, Grillflame, Centerlane, Starburst and Stargate.[10] It was run by Russell Targ, a physicist who was a pioneer in the development of the laser. He continued to work as a senior staff scientist at Lockheed Missiles and Space Company until 1997, having worked to develop airborne laser systems to detect air turbulence.

The pages in the now forgotten book which caught my attention were the ones that reported how outside the official RV programme, some of those who had been taught the skill of 'seeing' what was going on at a place and time removed from their physical bodies decided to 'visit' other planets in our solar system, which at that time had never been photographed. They gave detailed description of these planets, which later were proven to be highly accurate when the Hubble space telescope transmitted back pictures.

This apparently impossible feat attracted my attention and deep curiosity since it was conducted within the military establishment; not the sort of people usually associated with New Age psychology! Furthermore, the RV research was being conducted at the renowned SRI, under the control of a group of well-established scientists – well used to conducting experiments using a repeatable, verifiable protocol.

Intrigued, I read the published works of various members of the remote viewing team, *Psychic Warrior* by David Morehouse[11],

---

[10] Details of the CIA assessment of Stargate are provided in McMoneagle, Joseph. 1993. *Mind Trek, Exploring Consciousness, Time and Space Through Remote Viewing*. Chapter 7. Charlottesville, VA, USA: Hampton Roads
[11] Morehouse, David. 2000. *Psychic Warrior, the true story of the CIA's paranormal espionage programme*. UK: Clairview

Mind Trek by Joe McMoneagle quoted previously, *The Seventh Sense* by Lyn Buchanan[12] and *Limitless Mind* by Russell Targ[13].

The more I read the more convincing it became. These people have repeatedly produced accurate and verifiable descriptions and drawings of people, places and events located at a remote place or time. There are hundreds of examples accumulated over many years in a huge variety of circumstances, within the RV programme run by the military and after that, in the private enterprises that the remote viewers have set up, as well as in experiments conducted for television and film crews.

If this can be done, then the mind or spirit must be able to travel outside the physical body and through time. My rational brain recoiled at this, but the evidence presented in a scientific, lucid and rational manner seemed to be incontrovertible. There was only one thing for it; I had to find out for myself.

That was how I came to be sitting with over twenty other students in David Morehouse's 'Co-ordinate Remote Viewing' class in a beautiful countryside manor in Wales in November 2004. These students included several 'healers', two professional magicians who had basically come to de-bunk the whole thing and a number of serious and successful business people from a variety of professions, including myself.

The Co-ordinate Remote Viewing technique developed at SRI and taught by Morehouse is very prescriptive and methodical. It is a progressive, multi-stage, information acquisition process corresponding to increased contact with the target site that the viewer is being asked to visit and report on. It was designed to give information in a format that can be analysed and assessed through strict protocols, such that the output of several viewers looking at the same target can be combined to form a more comprehensive and cohesive picture. Features seen by a number of viewers gain credibility and different pieces of the jigsaw may

[12] Buchanan, Lyn. 2003. *The Seventh Sense, The Secrets of Remote Viewing as Told by a 'Psychic Spy' for the U.S. Military.* New York, NY, USA: Paraview Pocket Books

[13] Targ, Russell. 2004. *Limitless Mind, a guide to remote viewing and transformation of consciousness.* Novato, CA, USA: New World Library

start to fit together. In addition, some people are better at visuals, some at ambience, some at textures, some at sounds, some at motion and so on, so the summation of the output from a number of viewers can give a much more complete picture of the target than that given by one viewer alone.

The technique is that viewers are given a target to 'visit' and view which may be from any time period and anywhere in space. The target is identified simply by eight numbers starting with the current year (not the year which you are being asked to view) and then four numbers attached to the particular target being worked, whether that is a place, a person or an event, from massive to microscopic. These are not geographic co-ordinates but merely identifiers for the person directing the viewing. They serve no purpose except as labels for the site under observation.

There is a meditation based on Hemi-Sync sound[14] to guide you into the viewing. In the first stage when given a target, you are asked to give your immediate sense of 'the Gestalt': the overall impression presented by all elements of the site. To do this, on being given the eight digit identifier, you keep your pen on the paper and draw an 'Ideogram', the spontaneous graphic representation of the primary Gestalt. You then write down whether you think the target is natural or manmade, and whether it is a mountain, person, structure; is land, water or land-water interface.

Moving on from that initial impression you gradually consider colours, textures, temperatures, sounds, smells, size, energetics, aesthetic impact, motion, tangible factors, intangible factors and so on. The critical thing when remote viewing a target is to describe only what you feel, what you smell, whether it's hot or cold, the materials – what colour are they, are they

---

[14] Hemi-Sync sound is a Robert Monroe patented product which works by putting sounds of slightly different frequencies, known as binaural-beats, into the left and right ears. The brain then attempts to make a coherent whole from these vibrations, which results in the left- and right-hand side of the brain working together in unison, unlike normal activities which are conducted by one side or the other. Much more information about Monroe and his institution is given in Chapter 5.

rough or smooth, wet or dry? What is your sense of the size – is it vast or sub-atomic? What is the emotion you sense – is the location happy or sad, religious, evil, good, bloody, sacred and so on. It is totally experiential, not intellectual and you are using your senses, not your mind. You are encouraged to move around the site, to see things from different perspectives, to zoom in and out, and to experience what is there. At the end of each session you are asked to produce a written summary about your perception of the target.

What you must not do and what the logical, rational mind just loves to do, is to try to guess the actual identity of the target. This is called Analytic Overlay (AOL) and is almost certain death to a successful outcome. Of the options available throughout space and time, the locations you have in your head are but a miniscule subset of the locations you could have been sent to. But as soon as you think you know the answer, your logical mind will take over and construct a story, and you will no longer provide any useful information as a remote viewer.

In his teachings, Morehouse describes the AOL process as being when the mind jumps to one of a number of instantaneous conclusions about the incoming information without waiting for sufficient information to make an accurate judgement. This process is completely reflexive and happens even when it's not desired by the individual involved. Instead of allowing a holistic, right-brain process to assemble a complete and accurate concept, the analytic processes of the left-brain seize upon whatever bits of information seem most familiar and form an AOL with them.

A graphic example of the way that AOL can lead people off track was provided early in the course. The target that was set was actually Mount St Helen's volcano as it was erupting. Several of the viewers however were convinced they had been sent to the World Trade Towers on the 11th September 2001. They described heat, smoke, falling rocks, fire and so on, and then their logical mind took over and created a story about being in the Twin Towers. However the basic sensations they described were absolutely correct, they **were** viewing the volcanic eruption of Mount St Helen's, until their 'story' took over. During this particular viewing exercise, I had the vision of being on a mountain side beside a little cottage and a beautiful running stream. It is impossible to verify, but I may well have been at the right place, on the wrong date, prior to the volcanic eruption.

Over the space of six days we were taught the technique in stages and were given a variety of targets. And it worked! We were all beginners, unsure of this amazing journey we were embarking on, distracted by the group psychology, beset by doubt about our abilities, and exceedingly prone to the above mentioned AOL perennial problem that besets even experienced remote viewers. But it worked. I know that I perceived and experienced highly significant features whilst viewing at least two of the targets I was asked to visit and observe, simply through the use of the eight digit identifier. Out of all the millions of possible places in time and space I could have described, I got critical sensations pertaining to the targets I was being asked to view.

One of the instances that convinced me was when I perceived a black marble fountain. There were lots of buildings around with many arches in their frontages and also a tower. I then convinced myself that the target was Stanford University (which Morehouse knew well, but which he would not have expected any of his British audience to recognise. However I had taken my Masters Degree in Economics at Stanford from 1982 to 1984).

The actual target turned out to be the Kabala at Mecca, the sacred black marble stone set on water. There are lots of arches leading into the Medina and prayer minarets all around.

That was the moment when I knew without a doubt that somehow a part of me had been there, although my body was sitting in a room in Wales. There were just too many similarities out of the multitude of descriptions I could have given for it to be a coincidence.

How this worked I could not explain. But I knew from personal experience that it did. And once I had that knowledge, my world of cynicism and disbelief in the spirit, the soul and psychic viewing was turned upside down forever.

What I was forced to acknowledge as a result of these RV experiences is that **I am more than my physical body**. I had huge resistance to organised religion and any form of spirituality as a result of my childhood upbringing, so that was not an easy acknowledgement for me to make. Today I still have great anger about the way religion is mis-used in the world for power and control, and I certainly don't believe in any heaven or hell beyond those we create for ourselves in our lives on this planet. So this is a story about the science of our interconnectedness and ability to travel outside conventional space and time, initially driven by my experiences and then validated by my scientific reading. It is not a story based on any religious teaching.

So, what is it that is more than our physical bodies? Energy? Soul? Spirit? God? Consciousness? Information? These terms are used in so many different ways by people with different agendas. It may sound like semantics to worry about this but I increasingly see that really clear definitions of what we mean by some of these terms is critical to communicating about modern science, biology, philosophy and healing. In day to day conversations we simply don't have the language to express some of the difficult concepts I will cover in this book in a way we can all understand. We think we are communicating, but we are actually talking at cross-purposes.

Today, Remote Viewers continue to work across a wide variety of educational and investigative fields, for the wider benefit of humanity. Joseph McMoneagle continues to teach remote viewing at The Monroe Institute in Virginia. David Morehouse teaches a variety of Remote Viewing classes, including some aimed specifically at the medical profession or law enforcement officers. Lyn Buchanan runs the Assigned Witness Programme and works with police departments in the investigation of major crimes including missing persons, robberies, drug enforcement, gang activities, fraud and 'cold' cases, as well as working in the archaeological arena and with corporations in the area of counter-industrial espionage, problem solving, business planning and research and development.

Not surprisingly perhaps, we don't hear much about this in the media or our educational systems or our day-to-day lives. Nevertheless, thousands of people around the world have now been taught to Remote View and you may well have friends or colleagues involved in this growing movement. It's just that many people are not yet prepared to 'come out' regarding such experiences, which are beyond the limited mind conditioning that many of us have been brought up to believe in.

Chapter 3:

The Matrix, Non-locality and Quantum Entanglement

'Quantum physics is a new model of reality that gives us a picture of the universe. It is a picture in which many concepts fundamental to our intuitive understanding of reality no longer have meaning.'[15] (Stephen Hawking)

Some of you may have found the previous chapter difficult to believe. As I was experiencing the events described, so did I! What I was going through at the remote viewing course and subsequently was in complete contradiction to my belief system. Since I couldn't deny the experiences, the only rational conclusion was that I had to change my belief system.

My enquiring, journalistic mind was desperate to understand what was happening and come up with a rational, scientific explanation for the new belief system I was being forced towards by events, so I turned to quantum physics.

The theories of quantum physics are beautiful but complex and include concepts that often seem to defy 'normal logic'; however, their predictions and outcomes are most accurately

---

[15] Hawking, Stephen and Mlodinow, Leonard 2010. *The Grand Design.* p.68 London, UK: Bantam Press.

supported by experimental evidence. Even Albert Einstein, the father of general relativity theory, famously denounced quantum physics as a flawed theory back in 1935, saying it inferred bizarre and nonsensical concepts such as 'spooky action at a distance',[16] whereby particles were somehow 'entangled', allowing them to 'communicate' instantaneously with each other over vast distances. This seemed to contradict Einstein's theory that nothing could travel faster than the speed of light, hence he concluded that quantum physics had to be wrong.

Over the past several decades, some of the most modern and technologically advanced experiments conducted in linear accelerators have proved Einstein wrong and quantum physics correct. But even the best quantum physicists on the planet, including those that design and run these experiments, can often only **report** their results, without truly being able to **explain** them. Professor Richard Feynman, a key pioneer of quantum mechanics, who won the Nobel Prize in Physics in 1965, is quoted as stating, *'I think I can safely say that nobody understands quantum mechanics.'*[17] Almost fifty years later, we appear to be not much further on, although we have a lot more experimental evidence to validate the mathematical theories and a lot more knowledge about the impact that quantum mechanics can have on our lives.

The world I am about to lead you through is a strange world of uncertainty, probability, microscopic proportions, many dimensions, non-locality, the holographic universe and quantum entanglement. I will define these terms in more detail shortly, but if you are not a quantum physicist this chapter will probably be hard, as it challenges the rigid cause-and-effect world of Newtonian physics trapped in three-dimensional time and space.

---

[16] Letter from Einstein to Max Born, 3 March 1947; *The Born-Einstein Letters; Correspondence between Albert Einstein and Max and Hedwig Born from 1916 to 1955.* Walker, New York, 1971. (cited in M. P. Hobson; et al. *Quantum Entanglement and Communication Complexity (1998).* pp. 1/13.)

[17] Hawking, Stephen and Leonard Mlodinow. 2010. *The Grand Design.* p.74 London, UK: Bantam Press

This is what we live by and which we commonly assume is all there is to 'reality'. If you are a quantum physicist, apologies for my simplistic approach to what is undoubtedly one of the hardest subject matters on the planet!

If you just want the punchline, I have tried to summarise the conclusions and why they matter immediately below. That's followed by the theory and scientific evidence underpinning these seemingly improbable but scientifically proven conclusions.

Summary and so what?

The following are now accepted within the field of quantum physics as facts about what happens at the sub-atomic level. Knowledge of these facts is necessary in order to follow the rest of my story, even if you don't quite understand why they are true.

1. Quantum theory requires non-continuity, non-causality and non-locality. That is sub-atomic particles seem to disappear from one place and reappear in another place without following any one, specific path in between. This means we cannot know what happened in the past from observing the present. And things do impact on each other through 'spooky action at a distance'.
2. Nothing is known with certainty until it is observed. At the point of observation, the probability function of all possible outcomes 'collapses' into a measurable, actual event.
3. The act of observation itself impacts the outcome of everything that happens, from the behaviour of a photon travelling through a slit in a screen to whether someone is healthy or sick, in ways we still don't fully understand.
4. Non-locality has been demonstrated, suggesting that information is either the one thing that **can** travel faster than the speed of light, or is somehow 'just there', omniscient and omnipresent.
5. When applied on a large scale to the universe, the metaphor of the holographic universe suggests that each region of space-time contains information about every other point in space-time.

For me, as my story goes on to demonstrate, accessing this comprehensive information outside the 'normal' reality of linear time and space, is exactly the intention and function of altered states of consciousness, out of body experiences, remote viewing, shamanic journeying and so on. Metaphorically we have to become like the right light source which is required to read any hologram, which means sending out the right waves to access the holographic universe.

If you want to return immediately to my story and personal experiences, feel free at this point to jump straight to Chapter 4. But I really ask that you try to stick with me, for much of the theory that follows to justify the conclusions that I draw above is already fully accepted and well understood by physicists around the world and may transform how you view and experience the world around you.

Quantum physics and non-locality

One man whose life was changed by an acknowledgment of the implications of quantum physics is Dr. Bruce Lipton, a cell biologist who became a tenured faculty member at the University of Wisconsin, School of Medicine, internationally recognised for his research on cloned stem cells, before moving to Stanford University's School of Medicine. He is one of the leaders in the recently developed biology of epigenetics. He describes how as a medical student he ignored quantum physics, and continued to do so until a long flight, when he bought a book called *The Cosmic Code*, by Heinz Pagels[18]. '*Before boarding the plane in Chicago, I had no idea that quantum physics was in any way relevant to biology, the science of living organisms. When the plane arrived in Paradise, I was in a state of intellectual shock. I realised that quantum physics is relevant to biology and that biologists are committing a glaring, scientific*

---

[18] Pagels, Heinz. 1982. *The Cosmic Code:Quantum Physics As the Language of Nature*. New York, USA: Dover Publications Inc.

error by ignoring its laws... Biologists almost universally rely on the outmoded, albeit tidier, Newtonian version of how the world works. We stick to the physical world of Newton and ignore the invisible quantum world of Einstein, in which matter is actually made up of energy and there are no absolutes. At the atomic level, matter does not even exist with certainty; it only exists as a tendency to exist.' [19]

The next pages attempt to lead you through the concepts you need to build an understanding of the non-locality that appears to be central to quantum physics. This non-locality in turn opens the way to psychic phenomena as well as distance healing, energy healing and the power of intention (often called prayer) to influence the health of others as well as allowing us to be significant co-creators of our own destiny.

Holographic description of the universe

During the Remote Viewing course that I attended, David Morehouse explained that he believes Remote Viewing takes place by connection with a non-material and non-local 'Matrix' (and yes, this terminology was coined before the Hollywood blockbuster movie series).

The 'Matrix' itself is a huge, non-material, highly structured, mentally accessible framework of information containing all data pertaining to everything in both the physical and non-physical universe.

The simplest metaphor for the 'Matrix' from everyday language is the 'holographic description of the universe'. This term was coined by David Bohm, a theoretical physicist, in an attempt to explain the key evidence demonstrating that we can be affected by events that are distant from us in both space and time.

So what do we mean by a 'holographic universe'? This

[19] Lipton Ph.D., Bruce H. 2005. *The Biology of Belief.* p.68 : Carlsbad, CA, USA: Hay House, Inc.

concept is based on the hologram – a three-dimensional image displayed on a two-dimensional surface, which appears to move when you tilt it, or walk past it. The really bizarre thing about a hologram is that even if you smash it into millions of pieces, each tiny piece still incorporates the entire three-dimensional picture represented in the whole structure, totally unlike a conventional jigsaw. Each part of the smashed hologram will show the object from a different perspective as if you are moving around it, but it will include the entire object. In other words, a seemingly small, incomplete and disconnected piece contains within it the entire information of the big picture.

We probably all encounter holograms every day as they appear on all bank notes, credit and debit cards. So how are they constructed?

Lasers produce monochromatic light; that is, light of just one wavelength and hence one colour. This is different to most light sources such as the sun, desk lamps and camp fires which emit light consisting of many different wavelengths and colours. Lasers are also unique because they are 'coherent', which means that all of the peaks and troughs of the waves are lined up and move in sync, or 'in phase'. The waves line up spatially, across the beam, as well as temporally, or along the length of the beam.

To create a hologram, a laser sends a beam of light to a splitter, which splits the beam into two separate streams. One beam, known as the **object** beam, reflects off the object you want to represent in the hologram and onto a high definition photographic plate. The surface of the object is rough on a microscopic level, so it causes a diffuse reflection, scattering light in every direction. This diffuse reflection is what causes light reflected from every part of the object to reach every part of the holographic plate. The other beam, the **reference** beam, hits the same photographic plate without reflecting off anything other than a mirror.

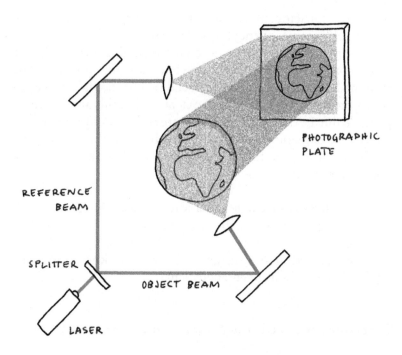

REFERENCE
BEAM

PHOTOGRAPHIC
PLATE

SPLITTER

OBJECT BEAM

LASER

Since the beams were originally joined together and perfectly in step, recombining them shows how the light rays in the object beam have been changed compared to the light rays in the reference beam. You need the right light source to see the hologram, but when the appropriate form of light is reflected off the surface of the holographic plate it makes an image. Your eyes and brain interpret this as a three-dimensional representation of the object in question. So a hologram is effectively a permanent record of what something looks like, seen from any angle.

Implications of the holographic universe

When the concept of a hologram is applied on a large scale to the universe, the metaphor suggests that each region of space-time contains information about every other point in space-time. Accessing this comprehensive information about events happening at a different place and time from what we think of as here and now, is exactly the intention and function of altered states of consciousness, out of body experiences, remote viewing, shamanic journeying and so on.

I don't want to try to stretch the analogy too far, but metaphorically we have to become like the right light source to read the hologram, which means sending out the right waves to access the holographic universe. Scientifically, this appears to be possible due to the enfolded, implicate order of our universe[20].

Before explaining what is meant by enfoldment and the implicate order, we first need to look at three key tenets of quantum physics:

1. Everything is a particle and a wave (at the same time!)
2. Nothing is known with certainty, only as a probability function
3. 'Spooky action at a distance' is real (also known as non-locality or quantum entanglement)

Everything is a particle and a wave (at the same time!)

Everything in this universe (including light, energies and objects) is both a particle and a wave. This duality is what challenges our certain and rigid cause-and-effect view of the world. A particle is fixed, its existence in time and space is certain. But the position of a wave is not certain and it is more pertinent to talk about the probability of its position.

Einstein's Nobel prize in physics was awarded not for his famous theory of relativity, but for explaining the photoelectric effect, revealing that light is actually transmitted in small discrete packets of energy called photons. For simplicity's sake, when you see a light beam you can imagine that it is really trillions of tiny but discrete lumps of energy coming at you.

The really bizarre thing is that at a microscopic scale, these photons and other subatomic particles flip back and forward

---

[20] David Bohm coined the term implicate order. The word implicate is based on the Latin verb *implicare*, which means to infold, involve, entangle, entwine, inwrap.

between being particles and waves depending on how you are looking at them and whether or not you are measuring them. And when you are not looking at them they have the potential to be either and just haven't decided which!

Much of the evidence for this is based on a succession of 'double slit' experiments, where particles are fired at a screen with either one or two slits open and a photographic plate behind it. It sounds simple enough, but the results are totally counter-intuitive and unequivocally demonstrate that particles have 'knowledge' of their surroundings, including whether you are observing them or not. In turn their surroundings somehow influence the likelihood of the form and position they take. How do they know? Why do they care? The answers to those questions are still a mystery, yet the observed results are now known.

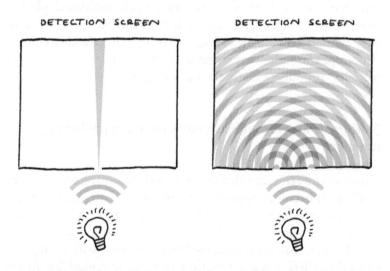

In the first experiment we consider a beam of light which is shone on a barrier with two vertical slits in it and a photographic plate behind. If just one slit is open then a single vertical strip of light is recorded on the photographic plate. If both slits are open, instead of getting two vertical strips you get a wave interference pattern. This is because light is primarily a wave (exactly like an ocean wave with highs and lows) – the dark circles are where two troughs meet and the light circles are where two peaks meet. This is typical of two waves interacting and you would get exactly the same pattern on water if you started two ripples a distance apart.

Since we now know that light is an electromagnetic wave, the interference pattern seems reasonable. Even though a light source is composed of many photons that are like particles, two of these photons can go through the two slits and interact with each other. Right?

Wrong! It turns out that when you turn the intensity of the light source down to fire just one photon at a time, the result is the same!

Conventional reasoning says that each photon must pass through either the left slit, or the right slit, producing a single dot on the photographic plate. This is what happens when only one slit is open and the photons are behaving like particles. But somehow, when both slits are open, each individual photon effectively goes through both the left slit and the right slit at the same time – interacting with itself to create an interference pattern. And repeating this experiment with electrons (microscopic particles) produces exactly the same results.

Nothing is known with certainty, only as a probability function

Quantum physics says that since all particles also have wave like qualities, it becomes impossible to pin down their exact location. There are an infinite number of possible positions which all exist at the same time.

This key concept is described mathematically by saying that everything has a wave function (a term invented by Erwin Schrodinger). The wave function tells you the probability of a particle being in a particular place at any given time. At the time of any actual observation of reality, whether in a physics experiment, or in life, the probability function of all possible outcomes 'collapses' into a measurable, actual event.

When the double-slit experiment uses electrons rather than photons, one electron is fired at a time towards the double slit, just in the same way as light photons were fired before. Prior to quantum physics we would have assumed that each electron is a particle, so we would have expected it to go through one slit – either the left one or the right one, and we would have expected to see two lines on the projection screen.

However, because the electrons have a wave like quality, their position is described by their wave function. This means that there are now an infinite number of places where each one might be found, no matter how improbable some of these places may seem.

The results of the experiment are the same as the experiment with the photons of light. The pattern produced suggests that each electron somehow 'knows' if both slits are open and the outcome is as though it went through both slits at the same time and interacted with itself. It is as though the electron travels every possible trajectory between its starting location and its final observed destination.

As Hawking describes this outcome, '*According to the quantum model, the particle is said to have no definite position during the time it is between the starting point and the endpoint. Feynman realized one does not have to interpret that to mean that particles take no path as they travel between source and screen. It could mean instead that particles take every possible path connecting those points. This, Feynman asserted, is what makes quantum physics different from Newtonian physics. The situation at both slits matters because, rather than following a single definite path, particles take every path, and they take them all simultaneously! That sounds like science fiction, but it isn't.*'[21]

Feynman also demonstrated something even more bizarre. If you **observe** which slit the electrons go through **before** they pass through that slit, then even with two slits open the interference pattern disappears! What you get are two parallel strips – what you expected in the first place when you assumed an electron to be just a particle.[22]

---

[21] Hawking, Stephen and Mlodinow, Leonard. 2010. *The Grand Design*. p.75 London, UK: Bantam Press

[22] Feynman went on to produce a mathematical construct known as 'sum-over-paths' which allows the motion of large objects to behave the way we expect in everyday life from Newton's laws of motion, whilst allowing microscopic objects, whose size is close to their wavelength, to take all paths between source and destination.

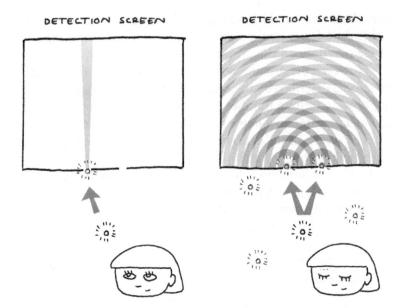

What this means is that by the act of observation the probability wave function breaks down and the electron is assigned a specific position in space and time. Now, through the act of observation there can be no question where the electron is. Physicists say that the wave function has collapsed, going from a state of an infinite number of probabilities to a state of one definite position. In this view, we, the observers, create the universe that we observe **through** our act of observation.

So, how do the electrons know how many slits are open? And how do they know if they are being observed? At present there are no definitive answers to these fascinating questions, so we have the empirical results but no proper theory to explain them.

Another implication of these experiments is that you will never know exactly what happened in the past if it was not observed. This means the unobserved past is indefinite – there is no exact one-to-one correspondence between cause and effect, so from observing the present we cannot draw any conclusions about what in the past caused the present we are now observing.

'Spooky action at a distance' is real (also known as non-locality or quantum entanglement)

As I noted above, in 1935 Einstein famously denounced Quantum Physics as a theory that was incomplete or flawed because it suggested that particles were somehow 'entangled' or interconnected with one another and could instantaneously communicate with each other over vast distances, challenging his hypothesis that nothing can travel faster than the speed of light.

Today the concepts of non-locality and quantum entanglement are widely accepted tenets of modern physics. Non-locality describes a way of entities being interconnected in a similar way to the metaphor of the hologram.

The physics underlying non-locality is a hypothesis known as Bell's Theorem as it originated from John S. Bell, who was a staff member of CERN (the European Organisation for Nuclear Research) whose primary research concerned theoretical high energy physics.

In 1964 Bell published the mathematical paper which transformed the study of quantum mechanics. **It showed that no physical theory which is realistic and also 'local' in a specified sense can agree with all of the statistical implications of quantum mechanics.** Many different versions and cases were inspired by this paper and are subsumed under the name 'Bell's Theorem'.

I will describe the details of the experiments which validated Bell's theorem below, but here is a short and metaphorical summary of it. Let's pretend you have two heads and four arms and standing back to back with yourself you throw two identical cricket balls in opposite directions at the same time. These cricket balls are spinning as they fly through the air, but we don't know if they are spinning clockwise or anti-clockwise. If we measure the direction of spin of one of these balls, then Bell's experiment shows that the other ball knows its twin is being measured and will make sure that it is spinning in the same direction – even though the probability of clockwise or anti-clockwise is 50:50. In other words, the two balls having the same source of origin (i.e. you) are inter-connected. In the language of quantum mechanics they are 'entangled' – exchanging information with each other instantaneously. This is what Einstein referred to as 'spooky action at a distance', also known as non-locality.

Dr. Abner Shimony, Prof. Emeritus at Boston University, wrote a long and highly technical article in the *Stanford Encyclopaedia of Philosophy* about the theory, the experimental evidence and the philosophy underpinning non-locality.[23]

As he explains, Bell's work followed on from earlier work by Erwin Schrödinger (1926) demonstrating that quantum mechanics permits entangled states, and a paper on non-casual correlations, known as the paradox of Einstein, Podolsky, and Rosen (1935) which *'examined correlations between the positions and the linear momenta of two well separated spinless particles and concluded that in order to avoid an appeal to non-locality these correlations could only be explained by "elements of physical reality" in each particle — specifically, both definite position and definite momentum.'*[24]

However, the uncertainty principle of quantum mechanics means that no definite position and definite momentum are possible simultaneously. So, since you can't define both the position and speed of each particle, you need to appeal to non-locality to explain the correlations between separated particles that are predicted by quantum theory. This was the paradox which led to furious intellectual debate for decades, until the experimental equipment to test the hypothesis became available.

The underlying experiment which finally resolved the theoretical argument about the existence or non-existence of non-locality was one in which two quanta of light, known as twins because they are ejected from a single source at the speed of light in opposite directions, are demonstrated to maintain their connection to one another, no matter how far apart they are. So

[23] Shimony, Abner, "Bell's Theorem", *The Stanford Encyclopedia of Philosophy*. (Winter 2012 Edition), Edward N. Zalta (ed.), http://plato.stanford.edu/archives/win2012/entries/bell-theorem/
[24] Shimony, Abner, "Bell's Theorem", *The Stanford Encyclopedia of Philosophy*. (Winter 2012 Edition), Edward N. Zalta (ed.), http://plato.stanford.edu/archives/win2012/entries/bell-theorem/

for example the measurement of the polarisation (direction of spin) of one of the photons determines the polarisation (direction of spin) of the other at its distant measurement site. If nothing can travel faster than the speed of light, as postulated by Einstein and at the core of physics for the last century, this measured result should be impossible. Yet it happens, demonstrating the existence of non-locality.

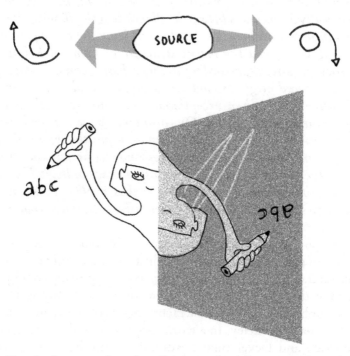

For the interested reader, Shimony describes a number of the major non-locality experiments at different centres around the world that have validated Bell's Theorem. At the end of his article he turns to the metaphysical conclusions of accepting non-locality.

One possibility is that, '*Yes, something is communicated superluminally*[25] *when measurements are made upon systems characterized by an entangled state, but that something is*

---

[25] Faster than the speed of light

information, and there is no Relativistic locality principle which constrains its velocity.'[26] In other words, as I understand this, information is one thing that **can** travel faster than the speed of light.

Shimony concludes, *'A radical idea concerning the structure and constitution of the physical world, which would throw new light upon quantum non-locality, is the conjecture of Heller and Sasin (1999) about the nature of space-time in the very small, specifically at distances below the Planck length (about 10^{-33} cm). Quantum uncertainties in this domain have the consequence of making ill-defined the metric structure of General Relativity Theory. As a result, according to them, basic geometric concepts like point and neighborhood are ill-defined, and non-locality is pervasive rather than exceptional as in atomic, nuclear, and elementary particle physics. Our ordinary physics, at the level of elementary particles and above, is (in principle, though the details are obscure) recoverable as the correspondence limit of the physics below the Planck length. What is most relevant to Bell's Theorem is that the non-locality which it makes explicit in quantum mechanics is a small indication of pervasive ultramicroscopic non-locality.'*[27]

As far back as 1975, the significance of non-locality and the ability of particles to communicate in a way that either breaks the rule on the speed of light being the maximum possible, or implies a connection with a source of information outside physical laws, was emphasised by physicist Henry Stapp of the University of California at Berkeley. In a work supported by the U.S. Energy Research and Development Administration, he wrote, *'Bell's theorem is the most profound discovery of science.'*[28]

---

[26] Shimony, Abner, "Bell's Theorem", *The Stanford Encyclopedia of Philosophy*. (Winter 2012 Edition), Edward N. Zalta (ed.), http://plato.stanford.edu/archives/win2012/entries/bell-theorem/

[27] Shimony, Abner, "Bell's Theorem", *The Stanford Encyclopedia of Philosophy*. (Winter 2012 Edition), Edward N. Zalta (ed.), http://plato.stanford.edu/archives/win2012/entries/bell-theorem/

[28] Stapp, Henry. 1970. *S-Matrix Interpretation of Quantum Theory*. Lawrence Berkeley Laboratory preprint, June 22. (revised edition: *Physical Review*, D3, 1971, 1303ff):CA, USA

The results of all this quantum theory are summarised thus by Bohm. '*Relativity theory requires continuity, strict causality (or determinism) and locality. On the other hand, quantum theory requires non-continuity, non-causality and non-locality. So the basic concepts of relativity and quantum theory directly contradict each other. It is therefore hardly surprising that these two theories have never been unified in a consistent way. Rather it seems most likely that such a unification is not actually possible. What is very probably needed instead is a qualitatively new theory, from which both relativity and quantum theory are to be derived as abstractions, approximations and limiting cases.*'[29]

And so, having investigated the holographic universe and the underlying tenets of quantum physics, I can finally move on to enfoldment and the implicate order.

Enfoldment and the implicate order

Bohm pointed out that until now the laws of physics have referred mainly to what he calls the **explicate order**, the normal, large-scale, three-dimensional world. He proposed that in the formation of the laws of physics, primary relevance has to be given to the **implicate order**, where we do not see a one-to-one correspondence between cause and effect and where each part of the universe contains information about the whole. The word implicate is based on the Latin verb implicare, which means to infold, involve, entangle, entwine, inwrap. So in some sense each region of the implicate universe, from the macrocosmic to the microcosmic, contains a total structure wrapped or entangled within it, as in the hologram.

Bohm describes enfoldment as the process by which a set of particles is spread out over such a large volume that their density falls below the minimum threshold that is visible. Unfoldment is the opposite, when the movement is reversed and the particles

[29] Bohm, David. 1980. *Wholeness and the Implicate Order*. p.223 U.K: Routledge & Kegan Paul

retrace their path to eventually regain their original, visible form. So the enfolded, microscopic world of many dimensions and non-locality has one set of rules, known to us as quantum mechanics, while the unfolded, macroscopic world of three dimensional day to day life has a different set of rules, defined by relativity theory. But it is the same particles that obey the two different sets of rules at different times, depending on how spread out they are and whether they are manifesting in our three dimensional world.

Thus Bohm proposes that *'The implicate order has its ground in the holomovement which is, as we have seen, vast, rich and in a state of unending flux of enfoldment and unfoldment, with laws most of which are only vaguely known and which may even be ultimately unknowable in their totality. Thus it cannot be grasped as something solid, tangible and stable to the senses (or to our instruments). Nevertheless... the overall law (holonomy) may be assumed to be such that in a certain sub-order, within the whole set of implicate order, there is a totality of forms that have an approximate kind of recurrence, stability and separability. Evidently, these forms are capable of appearing as the relatively solid, tangible and stable elements that make up our 'manifest world'. The special distinguished sub-order indicated above, which is the basis of the possibility of this manifest world, is then, in effect, what is meant by the explicate order.'*[30]

Can I explain this in really simple language? The truth is that no, I cannot. We are dealing with a description of an underlying 'reality' to the universe that we live in that in many ways defies our normal three-dimensional perceptions of space and time.

The best attempt that I can make is that what we perceive in our three-dimensional world is what Bohm describes as the explicate order. However this is just a small part of the larger multi-dimensional implicate order that underlies the explicate order and ultimately allows the things we perceive to work (this limited area of normal perception maybe why relativity theory

---

[30] Bohm, David. 1980. *Wholeness and the Implicate Order.* pp235-36 U.K: Routledge & Kegan Paul

works a lot of the time). However, the larger implicate order has to exist for quantum theory and the previously explained three tenets to be explained, including non-locality. The reason why we don't see the other underlying dimensions of the implicate order in our observed explicate order is explained by the second tenet in that we collapse the infinity of paths of particles into our 'reality' through our attempts to observe the universe.

In the Appendix to Chapter 6 of *Wholeness and the Implicate Order*, Bohm puts the notions of implicate and explicate order in a mathematical form. Interested readers are referred to the original work, which I am not qualified to replicate here.

Alternative visions

It should be noted that not all quantum physicists agree with the mathematical model put forward by Bohm. For instance, in *Limitless Mind*, Targ explicitly connects non-locality to our ability to view remotely and to psychic phenomena, with the non-local universe available to be accessed at will. The key to this access appears to be simply our intention. When we ask to receive information from the Matrix, we get it.

However, he has a different mathematical explanation of the non-local universe from that proposed by Bohm. He explains the ability to access information non-locally as the result of an apparent zero-separation between the viewer and the target within an eight dimensional 'complex Minkowski' mathematical model of space-time. In such a model, *'Each of the familiar three spatial (distance) and one temporal (time) coordinates is expanded by two into their real and imaginary parts... The complex eight-space model can always provide a path (the 'world line') in space and time that connects the viewer to a remote target so that the viewer experiences zero spatial and/or temporal distance in the metric.'*[31]

---

[31] Targ, Russell. 2004. *Limitless Mind, a guide to remote viewing and transformation of consciousness.* pp9-10 Novato, CA, USA: New World Library

In this view psychic phenomena are not the result of an energetic transmission and their description will not be found in electromagnetic fields, but are rather an interaction of our awareness with the **geometry** of the non-local, hyperdimensional space-time in which we live.

More fundamentally, the school of Relational Quantum Mechanics (RQM) takes a more radical approach. I met Professor Michel Bitbol at the Connecting Fields conference in Copenhagen in 2013 and I am indebted to him for bringing this alternative philosophy to my attention.

Having qualified in both physics and philosophy, Bitbol now focuses on the relations between the philosophy of quantum mechanics and the philosophy of mind and consciousness. As he explained to me, experiments validating Bell's Theorem show that quantum mechanics violates a *'realistic local theory'*. The usual assumption is then to abandon locality. However, the RQM physicists argue that rather than abandoning locality, it is scientific realism that should be entirely relinquished!

Matteo Smerlak and Carlo Rovelli give a full explanation of the theory and the philosophical implications of this radical approach. As they say, *'the philosophical implications of RQM, especially for what concerns realism, are heavy.'*[32]

The relational approach claims that the notion of an objective, absolute, 'state' of a physical system, or the notion of an absolute, real, 'event' are unjustified. The basic premise is that the observer and the event they are observing are tied inextricably together, so different observers can give different accounts of the actuality of the same physical property or event. This implies that the occurrence of an event is not something absolutely real, but is real **only** in relation to a specific observer. Thus quantum events are assumed to exist only in interaction with and relative to the system involved in the interaction and so my observation of an event and your observation of an event cannot simply be juxtaposed – they are independent.

---

[32] Rovelli, Carlo, and Smerlak, Matteo. 2007. 'Relational EPR', *Foundations of Physics.* pp37: 427–445

Epistemology is the study of knowledge and justified belief.[33] It raises questions such as what are the necessary and sufficient conditions of knowledge? What are its sources? What is its structure, and what are its limits? How are we to understand the concept of justification? What makes justified beliefs justified? Is justification internal or external to one's own mind?

The RQM physicists and philosophers such as Professor Bitbol believe that quantum mechanics led to the collapse of the classical scientific paradigm, but the time has now come to challenge the classical epistemology too. *theory of knowledge*

I don't fully understand the relational approach, but what I simplistically take from it is that if I were to adopt that approach, I would create a view of the world entirely based on my own experience. This experience would still validate all my current shamanic and energy healing work but this philosophy would separate me from the majority of my clients and readers who still hold onto the classical assumption of an objective reality. So whilst acknowledging that the RQM model **may** be founded within a deeper philosophical truth, at least as an interim step this book 'explains' my experiences through the vehicle of non-locality, rather than non-realism.

Consequences

What I know from my own experiences is that somehow, as a result of non-locality and the holographic universe, I and many other healers, meditators, psychics and clients, **can** access the field, the Matrix, the cosmic ocean, the universal life-force, the implicate order, consciousness, the Source, the One, the Divine, God: whichever label your philosophy prefers.

Although this might seem far-fetched, the knowledge provided by quantum physics appears to be the start of the rational explanation of how this can occur.

If you choose to, will to, intend to – then you too can get in

---

[33] Stanford Encyclopedia of Philosophy,
    http://plato.stanford.edu/entries/epistemology/

touch with the holographic universe, with potentially enormous benefits for your health, your relationships with other people and your relationship with the planet that we live on.

Chapter 4:
Rebirthing – Opening the Door to the Eternal Self

'Learning is limited. Learning can awaken your head but not your heart or your soul. Some of the most learned people I know are the least wise. They know too much and understand too little. Feeling, experiencing, doing – these are the acts that change our lives. These are the acts that pierce heart and soul.'[34]
(Dr. Dharma Singh Khalsa and Cameron Stauth)

24th April 2005. Little did I know when I woke up, how important this day would be. Initially it was one of those scary days which could potentially have put me off any further experimentation with altered states of consciousness, but as time passed after the initial event, it turned out to lead me to one of the most significant mentors and teachers of my life, for whom I still have great gratitude and huge respect.

I had an appointment to see a well known 'rebirther', Deike Begg, for a session at eleven o'clock. An acquaintance, Sean, whom I had met at the Remote Viewing course the previous November, had recommended her and the rebirthing process as

---

[34] Singh Khalsa, M.D., Dharma and Stauth, Cameron 2001. *Meditation as Medicine.* p.261 New York, NY, USA: Fireside

something that would be beneficial for me on my path of Self-exploration and he was going to meet me afterwards for lunch.

In her book, Deike defines the rebirthing process as follows, *'In Rebirthing you are taught how to consciously connect to your soul by connecting with spiritual energy and drawing it inside yourself with the breath. The effects of this are immediate and permanent. Every little step of progress is irreversible and every little step is an initiation for the soul. Essentially, Rebirthing is a breathing therapy in which you consciously connect to the divine power of the universe so that it will cleanse and transform you.'*[35]

Having read books on rebirthing and having heard from Sean of his experiences with the technique, I was interested to see how such a simple process could apparently impact people so significantly and so quickly. I later learned that breathing in a variety of ways to alter our consciousness is a technique that has been known to yogis for thousands of years, but has only recently been validated in the Western medical world.

As Roger Woolger writes in the Foreword to *Rebirthing*, *'The techniques of Rebirthing and recalling past lives were naturally known to ancient yogis and shamans the world over, but they were not widely taught to most people. Today we are once more being given these powerful tools and regaining a fuller understanding of the human psyche and its higher states of consciousness so that we can purify the agonies of our unfortunate birth circumstances past and present, and release the traumatic residues of abandonment, violence and premature deaths from past lives.*

'All such residues are imprinted in the subtle body or energy field that 'descends' into matter at conception to 'programme' our present karma at every level down to the cellular. These karmic patternings become the unconscious psycho-spiritual blueprints for our lives and determine our psychological development, our health patterns and our fate in general. Heavy accumulation of unreleased or unresolved karmic patterns leads, when not made

---

[35] Begg, Deike. 1999. *Rebirthing, Freedom From Your Past.* p.13 London, U.K.: Thorsons

44

conscious, to difficult births, tragic life stories, addictions, disease and 'all the heartache and the thousand natural shocks that flesh is heir to'.[36]

Anyway, so much for the theory – it was the practice that once again convinced me much more than any book.

I turned up at the mews house in Kensington that Deike was using for her individual rebirthing sessions that day. I remember walking in and up the stairs and talking to her about astrological charts and moons and phases – all terms that I was completely unfamiliar with and not what I had been expecting at all – I thought I was going for a breathwork session – not an astrological reading. Then I remember lying down...

The next thing I remember was finding myself in Kensington Gardens, with Sean beside me. I was walking on the grass in my bare feet and he was carrying my shoes. Why was I here? What had happened? What time was it?

It was two pm, and the last three hours of my life had completely disappeared from my memory.

Apparently, I had started breathing, guided by Deike, and then I had gone into a deep breath suspension and an out of body experience. She had not been able, during the limited time session before her next client, to get me to come back to physical reality. Deike to this day remembers it as one of the most unusual sessions in her long career as this very rarely happens! My spirit was off in another dimension, although I still have no recall of where I went. Her interpretation was that I had regressed into a previous life, where I had suffered a blow to the elbow and an accident of some sort that had left me unconscious and probably in a coma that I never recovered from. Somehow my mind had re-locked into the trauma of that coma, but I have no memory of what took place.

Sean, a healer with fifteen years of experience in Reiki and intuitive healing, had turned up to collect me from the session to be told that I had short term amnesia, but that the breathwork

---

[36] Begg, Deike. 1999. *Rebirthing, Freedom From Your Past*. Foreword pp ix-x. London, U.K.: Thorsons

45

process was to be trusted and I would come around to the present in good time. Meanwhile, Deike asked him to take over from her and stay with me until I came back to this reality.

Now up until this point, I had only met Sean three times since the Remote Viewing course where we had met. We had arranged to meet for lunch so I could give him feedback on the rebirthing session, as it was something he had recommended, being a client and friend of Deike's himself, and having worked with this process on numerous occasions.

Instead here he was, with a relative stranger who had apparently lost her mind, walking me round and round on the grass, trying to 'ground me' and reconnect me with who and where I was! I was periodically sticking my head through the railings surrounding the park, looking into people's gardens and repeating the same phrase over and over again, '*I don't know where I am – where am I?*'

Since leaving Deike's flat, Sean had managed to locate my car, parked several streets away and had brought me to the gardens. As an experienced rebirthing client and energy healer in his own right, he did trust the process, but began to get worried when, in addition to not remembering anything about the previous three hours (including where I had parked the car and whose house I had dropped my daughter off at), I could not remember where I worked, what I did, or a myriad of other fairly major longer term facts about my life. Meanwhile Deike was checking in with him about my condition and guiding him between every client.

Once I 'came round' and at least recognised where I was and who I was with, he gave me a piece of paper and a pen to start writing down the answers to the same questions that I kept repeating over and over again, as my recall of the answers lasted about two minutes before I started off on the same track again. From that point he would not answer the same question twice, but told me to look at my notes, and the act of writing and then reminding myself that I had already asked a particular question, began to stabilise my memory.

Amongst the notes I took was the statement, '*I have amnesia at the moment. It's a lesson to knowing what it's like not being in control. I am to trust the process for however long it needs to be. I am not to keep repeating that I am disorientated.'*

We then went for something to eat, during which time I kept asking questions and writing down the answers. The hot food and the grounding gradually worked sufficiently for me to go and collect my daughter and drive home with her. However, even by Monday at work, as Head of Corporate and Financial Communication for a major FTSE company, I was not functioning in a 'normal' way. I was sorting through my in-tray, out-tray and e-mails to figure out what I had and had not done.

Deike had been in touch regularly since I left her and because she had flown out of London as soon as she had finished her client appointments the day we had met, she had given me the number of her own teacher, Diana, another immensely experienced rebirther who lived and worked in London. She advised that I should see Diana as soon as possible to 'complete' the session.

I called Diana from work on Monday morning and quite frankly would have taken the rest of the day off as 'sick' if she could have fitted me in there and then. Unfortunately however she had no appointments immediately available.

My return to 'normality' and full remembrance of my everyday life actually came during the week when I went to my yoga class. During the yogic breathing my normal consciousness gradually returned. Retrospectively of course I wondered why on earth I had not thought of that and done a yoga session earlier, but at that time I was still thinking very conventionally and not in terms of synchronicities[37] or energetic patterns of behaviour. Interestingly, or I should really say synchronicitously, Deike herself is an expert on synchronicities and has written a whole book about the phenomenon.[38]

The following week, with some trepidation, having just 'recovered my senses', I went for my appointment with Diana, who was aware of the previous experience. She recognised my nervousness and took me very gently into the rebirthing breathing

---

[37] The Jungian definition of a synchronicity is a coincidence that has a personal meaning beyond the immediate facts of the situation.

[38] Begg, Deike. 2004. *Synchronicity: The Promise of Coincidence.* U.K.: Chiron Publications

pattern once again, reassuring me the whole time that I was safe, that it was safe to breathe and that she was there to help me.

On this occasion I did not lose consciousness at all, but had a wonderfully refreshing session. A lot of old painful topics did come to the surface and I had deep, rhythmic contractions in my stomach and pelvis as the breath entered my body and worked to clear old, stored memories and blockages.

Afterwards Diana gave me my first ever set of affirmations – positive statements of intent used to adjust your habitual thinking. Her way of working is to write each affirmation four times a day for a week, in the first, second and third persons. The lines she recommended for me were, '*It is now safe for me, Evelyn, to ask for what I want. It is now safe for you, Evelyn, to ask for what you want. It is now safe for her, Evelyn, to ask for what she wants.*'

I started these on Wednesday 4th May and finished a week later on 11th May, my forty-seventh birthday. On that day I wrote, '*Today is my birthday and today I don't need to write this anymore because I accept it.*'

Another commitment that I made on that day was to not ever again worry more about my public image and what other people think of me, than what I think of myself and what I know is important for my spirit and my wellbeing.

These may sound minor and insignificant steps, but they were huge energetic and psychological changes for me in my way of thinking and my belief system. Until that point I had often done things which didn't truly make me happy and which didn't even feel good, but I did them because of my fear of being judged by society. For instance, after I got divorced from my children's father I had very quickly bounced into another completely unsuitable relationship. I tried desperately to make that work for a prolonged period, despite the fact that I knew at a deep level it was not good for me, because I did not want to admit to my friends and my family that I had 'fucked up' again.

Because of my conditioning and the experiences I had had until then in my life, I had been scared of asking for any help or showing any vulnerability. I would have perceived that as weak and not acceptable. I was afraid of being judged and found lacking.

Now I can recognise that my fear stemmed from a lack of

self-love, but I had no knowledge or concept of that back then. Being able to step away from requiring societal and family approval of my actions, in an attempt to win conditional love, was the first step to respecting my own conscience, needs and purpose.

I went on to do numerous more rebirthing and psychotherapy sessions with Deike, who became an extremely important mentor and role model for me. She introduced me to several of the schools of teaching that I became involved with as well as leading me through a number of profound individual sessions where I came face to face with much repressed pain, anger and shame, which needed to be acknowledged and healed. Each and every session was quite different, displaying the power and diversity of experience possible through the rebirthing technique. However, none had quite the impact of that first session, which truly changed my life.

Chapter 5:
The Monroe Institute (TMI), Out of Body Experiences (OBE) and the Gateway Programme

'A condition where you find yourself outside of your physical body, fully conscious and able to perceive and act as if you were functioning physically – with several exceptions. You can move through space (and time?) slowly or apparently somewhere beyond the speed of light. You can observe, participate in events, make wilful decisions based upon what you perceive and do. You can move through physical matter such as walls, steel plates, concrete, earth, oceans, air, even atomic radiation without effort or effect... You can enter other reality systems only dimly perceived and theorized by our time/space consciousness.'[39] (Robert Monroe)

By May 2005, shortly after he had introduced me to Deike and looked after me during the initial aftermath, I had become Sean's partner, in the first stage of my sexual awakening, which is described in more detail in Chapter 13. Because we had met at

---

[39] Monroe, Robert A. 1985. *Far Journeys.* p.3 USA: Doubleday

the Remote Viewing programme and because of the close links between TMI and RV, a trip to TMI was the obvious next step for both of us, and we visited it together for the Gateway programme in April 2006.

Robert Monroe was a successful and distinguished business executive and noted pioneer in the investigation of human consciousness. For many years, he produced radio programmes and became well-known as a composer of musical scores for radio, motion pictures and television. His company owned and operated several radio stations and later, cable television systems.

His interest in human consciousness began in 1956, when he set up a small research and development division to study the feasibility of accelerated learning during sleep through the use of various sound patterns. He and his sound engineer researchers discovered they could create patterns of sound generating 'hemispheric synchronization'. 'Hemi-Sync' as it is known, is now a Monroe patented product and it works by putting sounds of slightly different frequencies, known as binaural-beats, into the left and right ears. The brain then attempts to make a coherent whole from these vibrations, which results in the left- and right-hand side of the brain working together in unison, unlike normal activities which are conducted by one side or the other.

Various electrical brain waves are known to be indicators of states of consciousness (such as awake or asleep). When you listen to a particular sound pattern the brain tends to resonate with similar electrical signals, and sound can therefore help you to be in a desired state of consciousness. With Hemi-Sync the whole brain is focused in an identical state of awareness at the same time and the condition can be changed at will by changing the sound pattern. Brain scanning machines can be hooked up to users of Hemi-Sync and they demonstrate the quite different brain wave patterns with and without the synchronisation.

Over many years of research Monroe and his colleagues tested many sound patterns and they discovered that certain patterns of Hemi-Sync sound resulted in people travelling out of the body, to different times and locations – most definitely not the original intention of their research!

The research division at The Monroe Institute (TMI) explains the ability to induce OBEs in physiological terms as follows, '*How we interpret, respond and react to information, is managed by the brain's reticular formation stimulating the thalamus and cortex, controlling attentiveness and levels of arousal. In order to alter arousal states, attentional focus and levels of awareness, it is therefore necessary to provide information input to the reticular activating system (RAS). Hemi-Sync provides this information, which is recognized by the RAS as brain-wave pattern information. If internal stimuli, feelings, attitudes, beliefs and external sensory stimuli are not in conflict with this information, the RAS will alter states of consciousness to match the hemi-sync stimulus as a natural function of maintaining homeostasis.*' [40]

His own out of body journeys were written up in a trilogy of books: *Journeys Out of the Body*,[41] *Far Journeys*[42] and *The Ultimate Journey*[43]. To develop this work he founded The Monroe Institute[44], which today is a worldwide organisation, headquartered in the rolling hills of Virginia USA, dedicated to expanding human potential.

In *Journeys Out of the Body*, Monroe warns would-be participants in OBEs of their life altering potential, a warning I re-iterate given my own RV experiences which set me off on such an unintended path with such wide-ranging consequences! He writes, '*Beyond this point (of physical disassociation), I believe you cannot turn back. Ultimately, you will be committed to the reality of this other existence. How this will affect your personality, your daily life, your future and your philosophies rests entirely with you as an individual. For once you have been 'opened' to this other reality, you cannot completely shut it out again, try as you might.*'[45]

---

[40] Atwater, F. and Holmes,Skip. 2004. *The Hemi-Sync Process.* USA: Research Division, The Monroe Institute

[41] Monroe, Robert A. 1971. *Journeys Out of the Body.* USA: Doubleday

[42] Monroe, Robert A. 1985. *Far Journeys.* USA: Doubleday

[43] Monroe, Robert A. 1994. *Ultimate Journey.* USA: Doubleday

[44] http://www.monroeinstitute.org/

[45] Monroe, Robert A. 1971. *Journeys out of the Body.* p. 215 USA: Doubleday

All I can add here is that for me that opening has been totally worth it. I am so grateful I was led to it and I would recommend it for everyone, although it may involve short term pain as we re-visit our repressed traumas, fears, shame, guilt and all the other karmic wounds we are carrying. The intention is clear – it is to release the negative impact of these wounds, freeing us to grow, evolve and truly step into our potential.

Monroe quickly got involved with the Remote Viewing programme being run out of the Stanford Research Institute (SRI) by Russell Targ and his colleagues. When news of his OBE experiments got out, the SRI team asked him to see if he could help Joe McMoneagle, one of the leading Remote Viewers, to get into the right state of consciousness to Remote View more quickly than otherwise. It soon became clear that Hemi-Sync was highly effective in this, so it became integrated into the RV programme.

McMoneagle became one of the most famous and best authenticated of the 'psychic spies' and to this day continues to teach and conduct his research at the Monroe Institute.

As an engineer, Robert Monroe was keen to find the scientific explanation for his out of body visits to other locations and his whole Institute was set up to run on verifiable, scientific principles. He describes how in one test a disassociation from the physical body was attempted from within a Faraday cage, where the physical body was completely surrounded by a strong direct current electrical field. Movement through the charged walls of the cage was impossible. With the charge removed there was no problem. This appears to suggest that consciousness can potentially be explained and rationalised scientifically in terms of the electro-magnetic field.

According to its website, since 1974 TMI has hosted programmes attended by over twelve thousand people. Its vision is to be a leading force for in-depth self discovery and transformation through research, education, enquiry and innovation. It is involved in hundreds of research projects into topics such as relaxation, meditation, stress reduction, pain management, sleep, healthcare, anaesthesia and the treatment of anxiety. The techniques pioneered there are also now being used in producing enriched learning environments, enhanced memory, improved creativity, increased intuition and telepathy.

The 'Gateway' programme that I participated in during April 2006 is a prerequisite to all the other more advanced programmes on offer at the Institute. In this programme, Hemi-Sync sound is used in conjunction with guided meditations, to help participants reach altered states of consciousness labelled 'focus levels'. These numbered focus levels are given to various defined states, simply because as human beings we communicate through language and we need labels that have a common meaning.

Prior to attending the course, participants are sent some preliminary 'homework' including a basic CD for the state of awareness known as focus ten. Try as I might, no matter how often I listened to this CD, I just could not stay awake! In focus ten my mind was supposed to be alert whilst my physical body was asleep. Now my unconscious mind may well have been awake and alert, but my conscious mind definitely checked out, so no matter what wonderful experiences I had whilst in focus ten, my recall was zero! As a result it was with some trepidation that I turned up at the beautiful TMI headquarters in the Blue Ridge Mountains of Virginia. We were all shown into our individual sound booths, where we would sleep and be guided through a succession of exercises moving to different focus levels over the next six days.

The instructors were at pains to reassure us that as they described it 'clicking out' (or as I described it, falling asleep) is quite normal, and that your subconscious gets the benefit of the 'journey' whether or not your conscious mind remembers, but my rational self wanted proof that I had been somewhere out of body rather than just sleeping for a week!

When I attended the Gateway programme, the group consisted of a variety of perfectly 'normal' people, from the USA, Canada, the UK, Germany and Holland. Their occupations ranged across a wide spectrum, including fire-fighters, a yoga teacher, a very well known author and several highly influential and successful businesspeople whose friends and families were completely unaware of where they were or what they were doing. Often the participants wanted to keep it that way for fear of being socially ostracised if people knew what they were going through and experiencing.

The striking thing about this group was the number of

people for whom out of body journeying was involuntary and had been continuing over a long period of years. And let me repeat, these were not stoned hippies, but highly successful professionals, for whom TMI provides validation that they are not alone in what they are experiencing. They are not mad, nor are they in need of psychiatric counselling. In fact they are incredibly gifted and blessed, and as with any other skill, just need to learn how to use it properly.

The Gateway programme goes as far as 'focus twenty-one', defined as the bridge between the worlds of the living and the dead, where we can ask for guidance from beings of a higher vibrational frequency.

Each individual gets something quite different from the Gateway programme. I 'clicked out' quite a lot, but gradually as the week progressed and I combined the Hemi-Sync guided meditations with a rebirthing breathwork technique learned from Deike, I was able to have a couple of experiences that again convinced me this was real and not just the result of an over-active imagination.

In the group circle held after each exercise, others also described a variety of experiences, which for them were clearly as real as sitting in the room in Virginia and which gave them great emotional and spiritual comfort and support.

I also learned that I tend to experience things from the non-physical dimensions not through visualisation, but rather vibrationally. For instance I get strong energetic vibrations in my hands when I am healing but the energetic vibrations flow through my heart when I am looking for personal guidance. I was 'told' by the guides from beyond our physical world to learn to understand the vibrations better, to spend time experiencing and exploring them, feeling the energy centres and layers within and around the body.

On my first visit to TMI I wrote after one of the OBE exercises, '*it felt like I was being examined, like little bugs crawling up my arms.*' I also had many other experiences of 'other' hands working on my body and my energy field. For instance on one occasion after 'journeying' I wrote, '*I asked to meet my guides. I couldn't see anything so I tried to communicate a different way. Then my hands got very vibratory and hot, my heart started beating very fast. I got great pressure coming into my body. I realised my spirit guides will manifest to me through the energy vibrations rather than visually.'* On another occasion, *'I could feel the energy entities with my hands. I sense that I need to learn to understand these vibrations. I need to spend more time with them.'* Very similar sensations were to re-emerge later in my life in a completely different, shamanic setting, but they seem to be frequent experiences for me and many others as we get in touch with the energy field that surrounds us and of which we are a part.

A particular practical assistance and demonstration of the benefit of the information we can obtain from the Matrix came from one session at TMI where we were instructed to ask for guidance as we journeyed. I got a very clear message that I should put my house on the market when I got home, clear my debts and then have far more financial flexibility and less worry about making ends meet.

When I got back to London, I re-considered this 'message', but decided that although the large mortgage I was servicing was putting pressure on me each month, it was not sensible to sell up and that I was not going to take 'advice' from some spirit guide! I was not yet in a place of trusting the information that I received from journeying.

Two months later, completely by surprise, due to a change of senior management at my workplace, I was made redundant. Had I already sold the house, a huge weight would have been lifted off my mind. As it was, I had to face the fact that if the mortgage payments were to be met, I simply **had** to get a job paying at least as much as my old job, as quickly as possible.

Instead, as soon as I heard that I was to be laid off, I called in the estate agents and put the house on the market. I calculated that if I paid off all the debts I had, I would still have enough capital to invest and rent something reasonable from the income, or alternatively buy something smaller, owned by me rather than the bank, and still have cash in hand. Either way, selling up would take away all the worry and stress and enable me to consider a much wider variety of career options, potentially paying less but satisfying me more.

Once I had made that decision I knew in my heart it was right, and that I should have followed the message I had received at Gateway. It all just seemed to fit, cutting my expenses, having the ability to move into a more spiritually satisfying role than the financial communications work I had been involved in up to that point. The only mistake was not having acted on the guidance earlier, which would have allowed me to be in a better position by the time I was made redundant.

On another occasion during the same Gateway programme, I was given a number of messages whilst in an altered state of consciousness. These included:

- Everything I have done is OK, it is all part of my learning experience in this lifetime. I should stop beating myself up about some of the things I have done and I should stop feeling guilty. Just let go, it's as it's supposed to be.
- I should trust and move on step by step. Things will be all right and I will be shown. If I just trust and accept, opportunities will come up.
- One drop in a pond sends ripples throughout, setting up a whole wave motion, so take one step at a time and the consequences will materialise.

These messages have been reiterated to me by other teachers and circumstances in a variety of ways subsequently, but they were first revealed to me during the Gateway programme. They have been very challenging for me, and they have raised many fears about my financial security, but in my heart I know they are right. We cannot know what we will do tomorrow and what opportunities (or setbacks) will present themselves, so today we can only do what we think is right at this moment, without any real knowledge of what the future will bring. There is no point in living in the past and no point in focusing all our attention and energy on the future. The only place we can truly be present is now and the most we can do is to act each moment in what we perceive right then as being the best way possible.

Another profound experience I had, which taught me to be careful about accessing the Matrix, was shortly after leaving the programme. Sean and I were stopping off in New York on the way back to the UK, to have several days of holiday, sight-seeing and shopping.

On the first afternoon, when I was still not fully grounded in my body or back to 'normal' reality, we decided to go to the American Indian Museum in Manhattan. I lasted about ten minutes. Looking at some of the artefacts in the museum cases I somehow just knew that the museum labels were wrong. There seemed to be a very strong channel open between me and the time and place where a particular selection of the articles had been found. I could feel myself drifting to that location and I felt my head spinning as the sensations of that time swamped me. Sean could tell that I was losing control and I had to sit down before I fell down, so he managed to get me to a seat in the museum store while he continued to look around for another half hour.

I have no recall of that period, except being jolted out of it in a great fright as he came back and stood quietly in front of me. My mind had clearly once again left my body and visited another time and place. However my lack of control over the journeying process meant I couldn't recall the details.

We talked about needing to be in control of the OBEs and the energetic openings to and connection with other places and times. It is important to use them carefully, at suitable times and places, or else your current life could be over-run by too many sensations, images and thoughts crowding in from the people and objects around you, something that some sensitive psychics do suffer from and can be overwhelmed by.

It was another in the expanding variety of experiences which demonstrated to me that we are indeed more than our physical body and that our mind or spirit can travel beyond current physical reality. Some people travel spontaneously and are able to channel back in speech or writing the information they receive, but most of us need to be taught how to recall that information and use it judiciously.

Chapter 6:
The Monroe Institute and the Lifeline Programme

'We at TMI Research maintain that no one approach to the study of consciousness will suffice. We believe that only a multi-disciplinary, multi-voiced, multi-theory approach that includes open dialogue, collaboration, and a sharing of knowledge amongst colleagues (both professional and nonprofessional and from the many diverse areas of consciousness research) will provide true opportunities for gaining insights into the mystery of human consciousness.'[46] (Monroe Institute website)

I returned to TMI a second time in January 2007, this time by myself, to participate in what is called the 'Lifeline' programme. The experiences I had on this second occasion yet again challenged my rational mind but gave me profound insights and a really intuitive knowing that the story I uncovered during my OBEs is my truth, without which I truly don't believe I could be doing the shamanic work I am involved in today, openly and without fear.

Until this point I had read about past lives but I had had no direct experience of them. (During my first rebirthing session,

---

[46] http://www.monroeinstitute.org/research/overview-of-research-at-the-monroe -institute

Deike perceived that I had disappeared off into a past life, but since I didn't remember anything about that session, that didn't really count as a conscious experience.) That was about to change.

Many readers of course may not share my belief in reincarnation, past lives and karma but the concepts will recur repeatedly throughout the rest of this book, so I would like to very briefly address some of the religious, philosophical and scientific underpinnings to these now, before moving on in my story to take them as a given!

Reincarnation and karma

By human reincarnation I mean the persistence of a soul from one physical body to another over a succession of lives. By karma I mean the lessons, patterns and contracts we make with life, which we transfer between the succession of physical bodies we choose to inhabit.

For those who disbelieve in these concepts because they come from a Christian tradition, it is perhaps worth acknowledging that modern Christianity is almost unique amongst world religions in rejecting the concept of reincarnation. Billions of people across the world, including all Hindus and all Buddhists as well as most indigenous people, are brought up with this concept and find it entirely natural.

Based on the evidence uncovered within the Nag Hammadi library[47] it also appears that the original Christians and their followers (often known as the Gnostics), right through to the Cathars[48], did believe in reincarnation and considered the Old Testament god Jehovah to be a tyrant.[49] The Inquisition within

---

[47] The Nag Hammadi library is a collection of early Christian Gnostic texts discovered near the Upper Egyptian town of Nag Hammadi in 1945.

[48] The Cathar movement appeared in Europe in the 11th century and flourished in the 12th and 13th centuries. The movement was extinguished in the early decades of the thirteenth century by the Albigensian Crusade, when the Cathars were persecuted and massacred.

[49] Freke, Timothy and Gandy, Peter 2002. *Jesus and the Goddess, The Secret Teachings of the Original Christians.* p.71 London, UK: Thorsons

Europe was set up by the Literalist Christian Church specifically to eradicate the Cathars and these 'heretical' beliefs. Despite many persecutions the Gnostic free spirit was never entirely extinguished and indeed over the centuries it has inspired many of the great Western cultural heroes, including Dante, Leonardo da Vinci, Michelangelo, and most of the great minds of the Renaissance, as well as scientists such as Galileo, Copernicus and Kepler.

For those that disbelieve on atheist grounds, which is the place that I started my journey from, I totally accept that only a personal experience will convince you. All I can repeat at this stage is that as countless others have already discovered (most frequently, unintentionally, noticeably and dramatically through near death experiences), once you have had just one experience when you have **known** you are more than your physical body, your life will never be the same again.

Kenneth Meadows gives what I think is one of the best descriptions I have read of the journey of the soul from lifetime to lifetime. This particular description comes from the American Indian belief system, but uses amazingly similar language to that of Buddhist, Hindu and Taoist philosophies.

He writes, '*As the physical vehicle at death is cast aside, the Energy Body which is made up of fibres of energy in a web-like structure that links the physical with the more subtle planes, disintegrates. The Astral Body* [50] *then becomes the focus of the consciousness and in this body the individual is in a condition of awareness not unlike that experienced in Astral travel or shamanic journeying.*

'*After a period in this state, the Astral body breaks up and the individual progresses on through higher realms of awareness before the Circle turns and the individual begins the journey back to another lifetime, another birth, in a new physical body.*

'*With each new birth the Individuality develops a personality through which to express itself and through which to perceive life. The personality is therefore, transient too, being a by-product of a particular incarnation, and discarded along with the physical*

---

[50] The Astral Body is the field of energy that penetrates and surrounds the physical body.

61

body at death. The Individuality however, being immortal, survives, to continue its existence and its awareness.'[51]

He continues later, *'Each life then, was seen as a means of gaining knowledge and experience on a never-ending journey of self-awareness. Death was observed as not an end but a part of life – a vital element in the cycle of life, as night is to day and winter to summer, as the moon is to the sun. Death was a return to another plane of existence where the lessons learned from the lifetime just lived could be absorbed and understood and where the Individuality, after a period of rest, assessment and renewal, determined what was necessary for its continued development in the next lifetime.'*[52]

With such a belief system, what we do at any moment in time has implications for eternity as it impacts the story, the energy, the karma we carry into our next incarnations. Meadows' Native American teacher Silver Bear explained it like this. *'Our past lives have shaped our present destiny and brought us to the place in Time where we are now. Our present life, our present attitudes, will shape what we are yet to become.'*[53]

Lifeline

So, having digressed into reincarnation, back to the Lifeline programme at TMI, which is about moving to what it calls 'focus twenty-seven', or 'The Park'. Focus twenty-one is defined as being where the spirit departs from the physical body. Focus twenty-seven, also called 'The Park', is defined as being where spirits eventually end up to decide with their spirit guides and soul group where to go next, whether that is to be a reincarnation back into human form, or emerging as a different

---

[51] Meadows, Kenneth. 1990. *The Medicine Way, A Shamanic Path to Self Mastery.* p.112 Shaftsbury, Dorset, U.K.: Element Books Limited

[52] Meadows, Kenneth. 1990. *The Medicine Way, A Shamanic Path to Self Mastery.* pp112-113 Shaftsbury, Dorset, U.K.: Element Books Limited

[53] Meadows, Kenneth. 1990. *The Medicine Way, A Shamanic Path to Self Mastery.* p.113 Shaftsbury, Dorset, U.K.: Element Books Limited

type of energy or being. In between, focus twenty-two to twenty-six are different belief systems, known as bardo states, where spirits can get stuck for a prolonged period before moving on to The Park.

For instance if someone was in a heavy coma or heavily drugged before death, the spirit might already have partially left the body before the official time of death when the body completely ceases functioning. In such a case the spirit could have gone to level twenty-two or twenty-three. Energetically these are peculiar spaces, between life and death and when the physical body finally dies, the spirit may get stuck in this belief system for a while because it is not sure whether to finally leave the physical body.

According to Robert Monroe's own OBEs and journeys, as well as those of hundreds of those attending his courses, another example is that if people have a strong religious belief system during their lives about what will happen after death, such as they are sinners and will burn in hell, then they may indeed visit a bardo state that looks like their vision of hell for a while, before their spirit, out of the physical body and the societal conditioning, realises it doesn't actually need to stay there for eternity.

The intention of the Lifeline programme is to give participants the tools they need to travel out of body and then guide spirits from the various bardo states where they are stuck to The Park.[54] As it turned out however, for me, several days of the workshop were spent revisiting and resolving one particular past life of my own, which was holding me back from fully embracing the new path my life was taking.

---

[54] This is very close to the definition of a 'Psychonaut' that Robert Thurman gives in the *Tibetan Book of the Dead*, a very different tradition. He says a psychonaut is a voyager into the soul. He refers to the Buddhist adept who voluntarily abandons the pseudo-security of this planet of delusion, with its solid ground of ordinary, individuated suffering, to launch herself through the death-dissolutions into the subtle between-states to deepen her wisdom by exploring the unconscious and to expand her compassionate heroism by serving universes of beings on the subtle level, and then returns to the ordinary embodiment of the adept to assist her contemporaries.

Crucial re-writing of a soul contract

Up until the Lifeline programme, in this lifetime I had always been afraid of water and had hated swimming, particularly putting my head under water. As I went into an out of body state of consciousness for the purposes of a soul retrieval, guided by the Hemi-Sync, I revisited a previous life and death which involved being drowned as a witch. I could see myself tied to a chair, being lowered into a pond with a crowd around watching, including my daughter aged about ten or eleven. I could picture myself in that witch lifetime very clearly: I was a poor woman, with a long, tattered brown dress and apron and long brown hair tied up in a bun. I worked as a midwife and with herbs and plants, to make medicine for healing, not ill-use. For some reason that was not acceptable to the society I lived in and they accused me of being a witch. At that time of course if you did actually drown it proved your innocence, whereas if you didn't drown it proved your guilt, at which point you were usually burned instead. Whatever – the result was death.

Having re-experienced that death by drowning, from The Park I then had to go back to find that daughter whose name was Jessica. I learned that she had been sexually abused and effectively kept as a slave after I drowned, because she was the witch's daughter and no-one wanted her or cared for her. She died very young in childbirth and her baby, my grand-daughter, died too. After death, she went to a bardo state involving living in a cave in a forest, surrounded only by animals, the eagles, the wolves and the forest creatures. Her belief system was that she couldn't trust anyone, particularly men and just wanted to be by herself.

In my out of body consciousness, a spirit guide manifesting in the shape of a wolf helped me to find her, as he was able to guide me to the cave Jessica was living in within her bardo state and she would allow the wolf to approach, although she would have hidden from any unaccompanied humans attempting to enter her space. I eventually persuaded her to come with me to The Park, and she said she would come because she trusted me. That was an incredibly emotional experience for me when it happened because I did not feel as if I deserved her trust. It was my fault she had been so abused because she was the witch's daughter, yet here she was telling me she had faith in me.

One of the huge lessons that I got from this experience was that I made a soul contract after that lifetime, that *'From now on I will conform with authority'*. Soul contracts are something we write at times of deep trauma and wounding. We make a decision on how to live our lives in future to protect ourselves from the same wounding or trauma as that we have just experienced. These are not bad. They are contracts that we make at a particular time in an attempt to be safe and for a while they may well serve us.

In this particular instance, *'I will conform with authority'* was an attempt to prevent myself and the ones that I love from getting hurt again, in the way that happened in that witch lifetime. As a result, I have lived all my lifetimes since then doing what society has expected of me. And in living by that 'contract', I gave up who I really am. I lost my true self, the healer, the 'witch'. That realisation brought up a huge amount of emotion for me and a huge sadness, but also a huge release, because finally I could let that contract go, recognising it no longer serves me. The result was that I can reclaim who and what I really am, using the gifts I have been blessed with but which I have suppressed and ignored for so long.

All of these life-changing events gave me the knowledge that experiences in an altered state of consciousness can be just as 'real' to me as any in my 'normal' everyday life. It was not just like being in a dream or something happening in my imagination. I was not asleep, I was perfectly conscious, and indeed more alert than I am in much of my 'normal' life. It was like being in a movie and watching it at the same time!

Once again it confirmed to me that our spirits are not limited to the space and time occupied by our physical bodies, but can travel through and access information from the field, the Matrix, the enfolded or implicate order, the quantum sea of energy in which all things operate and manifest.

Healing the lineage experience 1

During the Lifeline programme I was also introduced to the concept of healing the whole lineage, the ancestors and the descendents, work that I have returned to since then time and time again, through shamanic healing, plant medicine, tantra and family constellations, a recently developed form of psychotherapy which involves standing in what practitioners label 'The Knowing Field'.

The basic concept is that even if our ancestors are now in a different physical body due to reincarnation, they may have karma from previous lifetimes stored within their energy field which can be released if I change my vibrational frequency and my thought patterns towards them. Scientifically this is again possible because of quantum entanglement and the fact that we are capable, with intention, of reaching through space and time when we enter the implicate order, the multi-dimensional holographic universe.

Alternatively, I may be carrying karma on behalf of a previous generation, which can be released by my actions in this lifetime. Thus we can heal past generations, seeing, acknowledging and honouring their suffering or their guilt, or even their atrocities. If necessary we can stop carrying their burdens and sickness on their behalf and pass these back to where they belong. This restoration and healing of the lineage can also pave the way for future generations to be free of ancient karma and curses.

Power animal links between TMI and Shamanism

In another premonition of the shamanic work to come, but not yet even conceived of, during one of my OBEs during the Lifeline programme I met eagle as a power animal. Many animals are recognised in different philosophies and tribes to have particular qualities and what are known as 'archetypes' are the representations of these qualities. Shamanism often calls in animal archetypes and spirits for the qualities they possess which may be of assistance to us in our lives at any given time. Eagle flies high, seeing the higher perspective, the bigger picture, wing to wing with the Great Spirit.

I recorded in my journal, '*Going out of body, I went into a dense, white fog where I was completely blind. I perceived a little girl of about twelve who took me by the hand and we went to talk to an eagle. Eagle told me to use my eyes for a different kind of seeing. Later in the same session hands were moved around my body to show me how to 'see' auras and feel the different energy centres. It didn't feel as if it was my own hands touching different parts of my body. It felt like the hands of my spirit guides. I saw the little girl and the eagle again as I was coming back into body and the eagle allowed me to touch its foot, but not its head.*'

I also felt the connectedness of all humanity. The easy way out is to ignore other people's pain and not get involved. It's not my problem. But in fact because we are all ultimately interconnected parts of the one universal consciousness, anyone's suffering **has** to be my problem and I need to offer whatever assistance I can.

Final lessons of Lifeline

One more lesson was just to trust and feel. I wrote in my journal at the end of the last exercise of the programme, '*I was told not to try to put things into words or even visualisations, but just to FEEL, sense the energy, use my sensations and my body, not my head. That's how I need to work. I got a huge sense of the fact that I am just energy, that I am supported and connected. I just need to stay true to my energy.*'

In my own personal journey, all these OBEs, past life experiences and lessons have been hugely influential in convincing me of the power of the non-local mind and our ability to access the Matrix.

If you don't believe in the universal energy field then none of the above is ever going to persuade you that you can journey out of your body or reach any of the potential altered states of consciousness, or get guidance from the superconscience under whatever label. I know and totally accept that only direct experience can ever change your belief system.

However, for those of you who are interested in scientific

validation, the research section of TMI's website[55] provides a huge amount of both quantitative and qualitative research conducted since 1956. I cannot possibly review the vast library of literature here, but I hope you will read some of the conclusions for yourself.

TMI itself has evolved over that period since 1956 and today one of its primary goals is an interdisciplinary approach to consciousness research, drawing together the findings from a wide range of thought-leaders across many fields, in an exemplary model of the generalist approach so lacking in today's world of narrowly defined specialisms.

As the website states, *'The question of what consciousness "is" and how it "works" is currently being approached from multiple perspectives. Philosophers, neuroscientists, psychologists, anthropologists, theologians, spiritual leaders, and practitioners of all kinds are all investigating questions regarding the nature and functions of consciousness through the specific lenses of their particular disciplines. At one end of the continuum are the materialists who argue that mental phenomena can be reduced to being a product of matter. According to this perspective, consciousness is not "real" in any independent sense but is instead the byproduct of physico-chemical processes. On the other side of the debate are the subjective idealists who, at their most extreme, regard mind as primary and matter nothing more than an illusion created by mind. In the middle are those who maintain that consciousness is the result of both physical and nonphysical properties, thus leading to the "problem" of (and resulting plethora of explanatory theories about) how these two phenomena "link up" to create subjective experience.'[56]*

I totally support this multi-disciplinary approach and this book is my attempt at a synthesis of the knowledge I have managed to glean from a wide range of experts and which I believe needs to be made accessible in an integrated package to inform everyone of their potential to access the superconsciousness and the information contained therein.

---

[55] http://www.monroeinstitute.org/research/overview-of-research-at-the-monroe-institute

[56] http://www.monroeinstitute.org/research/overview-of-research-at-the-monroe-institute Goal #3

Chapter 7:

Reiki – Universal Energy Healing

*'My colleagues and I trained our students to disregard the
healing claims attributed to acupuncture, chiropractic, massage
therapy, prayer etc... We denounced these practices as the
rhetoric of charlatans because we were tethered to a belief in
old-style, Newtonian physics. The healing modalities I just
mentioned are all based on the belief that energy fields are
influential in controlling our physiology and our health.'*[57]
(Bruce Lipton)

Two of the huge gifts I received from my two year long
relationship with Sean were an accelerated introduction to a
variety of forms of energy healing and an initial introduction to
my sexuality, which until I met him had been totally repressed
by my childhood conditioning.

Although he was a director of a sizeable company in the UK,
hence well grounded in the business world, by the time I met
him Sean had also been a Reiki Master and intuitive energy
healer for fifteen years. He was also training in shamanic and
Native American healing practices.

---

[57] Lipton Ph.D., Bruce H. 2005. *The Biology of Belief.* p.69 Carlsbad, CA,
USA: Hay House, Inc.

Within a condensed space of time, he introduced me to rebirthing, craniosacral therapy, shamanic healing and a variety of other energy healing practices, as well as giving me my first Reiki treatments and my Level 1 Reiki attunement. Together we went to the Monroe Institute for the Gateway course I have described already and later that year I visited him in Arizona where he was working with Native American healers. I owe him so much for turning my life-path around and seeing potential in me that I didn't know existed.

Reiki

Literally translated, Reiki means universal energy. It was transmitted to (or some would say rediscovered) by Mikao Usui in Japan early in the 20th century. Originally he handed his teachings down to a very small number of initiates or Masters. But in the last years of the 20th century a number of Reiki healers felt that the earth and humanity needed as much healing as possible and as many healers as possible, and decided to widen the number of those initiated or 'attuned' to the Reiki forces.

The five principles of Reiki are as follows:

- Just for today I will give thanks for my many blessings
- Just for today I will not worry
- Just for today I will not be angry
- Just for today I will do my work honestly
- Just for today I will be kind to my neighbour and every living thing

For those of you who have never experienced a Reiki treatment, it is usually, but not necessarily, a hands on method of healing, whereby the therapist starts at the crown of the head and works through certain energy centres, known as chakras (which are explained in much greater detail in the next chapter), down to the feet, connecting with the client's life force energy, at the physical, emotional, mental and spiritual levels.

There are three levels of 'attunement' to the Reiki energy. Level 1 gives you the ability for self healing, Level 2 gives you the ability to heal others and Level 3 gives you the ability to pass on the teachings to others, to be a 'Master'.

Sean gave me my first Reiki attunement in September 2005, almost a year after we had met at the Morehouse RV course. I had awaited this ceremony with anticipation for a number of weeks and he had asked me during that time to become vegetarian and abstain from alcohol, to detox my system and raise my receptiveness to the transmission I would receive. I actually discovered during that time that I didn't miss meat and fish at all and I have been vegetarian ever since then. I haven't given up on wine however!

Even though I had felt the power of healings he had already given me to release long held emotions (in particular, suppressed anger), my left brain was sceptical, but the attunement itself was very beautiful and powerful. There is a meditation which introduces you to your Reiki guide and then the Master puts the Reiki symbols into your crown chakra and your hands.

There are four principle symbols in the Usui Reiki tradition, which mean:

- Put all the power of the universe here
- God and humanity joined together in love, wisdom and harmony
- The God consciousness in me reaches out to the God consciousness in you, in love, wisdom and harmony
- Great being of the universe, shine on me, be my friend

Having received the Level 1 attunement to the universal energy, my dominant left brain still wanted proof that it worked before I went on to Level 2 for healing others. I believe that entirely to give me this proof, when I was skiing in Les Trois Vallees in France, in December 2005, I fell on Christmas day, and had to be carried down the slopes to the local hospital in the 'blood wagon'. The outcome of the fall was that my left knee was severely damaged, with ruptured medial and anterior cruciate ligaments (ACL), as well as significant damage to the cartilage in between.

My consultant at King's College Hospital in London was keen for my knee to heal as much as possible before he operated to replace the ACL – in particular he wanted the severe swelling to go down. That meant a ten week delay before surgery, during which time I did Reiki self healing on my knee every single day. Sean also worked with me when he could, using Reiki and hypnotism to bring in healing, and I was seeing a physiotherapist for exercises.

In March 2006 I had the surgery. When the consultant came to see me as soon as I came out of the anaesthetic, he expressed his total surprise. *'I have never seen anything like it! I did have to replace the ACL as anticipated, and that went well, but I didn't have to do any of the other work that I was planning for the medial ligament or the cartilage. They had healed themselves! I don't understand how, it's very unusual.'* I didn't bother to tell him how... but I had my proof.

Giving energy healing

A few months later, after receiving the second attunement, I started working with clients professionally and fifteen months later I was attuned to the Master level. Now working with Reiki energy has become part of my life and the profound healing for clients that results is astonishing. Each client continues to be my teacher, as each individual has their own life experiences, their own 'story' and their own belief systems. No two sessions are ever alike, even with the same client, and I never know where the Source, universal energy, Inner Physician or whatever you want to call it, is going to lead, and what the body and the energy system are going to present for healing on any particular occasion.

I do totally trust however that only clients that I can be of service to will turn up at my door. When I first started practising, I was sent people with relatively 'easy' problems. Those problems and issues were of course very painful for those clients and I in no way wish to belittle them. They were suffering from stress, relationship break-up, back injuries and so on. However, the individuals I saw initially did not present as being seriously wounded or damaged through chronic abuse or illness. They weren't suicidal or psychotic.

Of course I am a different therapist these days, so the systems of those same clients might now present more serious problems to me were I to meet them today, but as my practice has expanded and deepened, I now get some clients whose stories are truly traumatic. I often wonder how they are managing to function at all given what they have experienced. Yet they are frequently working very successfully in their professional lives, hiding their pain from their friends and colleagues and sometimes from their families too. But underneath the societal mask they wear, they have deep wounding and trauma, which is making them sick in a variety of ways and which the Reiki helps to release and transform.

When I am giving energy healing and bodywork, I work primarily with the chakras (the energy centres described in more detail in the next chapter), feeling for blockages, pain or imbalance. Once I have felt that there is a problem, I focus on whether it has a physical, mental or emotional cause. There is also the issue of the time frame associated with the problem. Is it relatively new or very ancient? Is it something that originated during the birthing process? Is it something brought in from a past life? Is it the result of a recent accident or trauma? Is it associated with pharmaceutical or recreational drugs? I simply ask the system and accept whatever answer comes to me.

Frequently when I work with new clients I know very little about their 'story'. The first time we meet I prefer to tune into their energy system and see what it presents for healing at that moment in time. It also builds far more trust with the client if I tell them what I feel and it resonates with them, rather than them having given me the information.

Over the years I have gradually learned to trust the sensations, images and words I get when I am working in this way. Sometimes the information may manifest as physical transference, in which case I get a physical pain that mirrors a pain of the client's. Other times I get a feeling of imbalance between the left and right-hand sides of the client's body, which often represents an imbalance in or conflict between the masculine and feminine parts of the person. It may represent a wounded feminine, for instance as a result of sexual abuse, abortion, hysterectomy and so on. Sometimes the information comes simply as words in my mind, a knowing that the client has a damaged immune system or suffered a traumatic birth, that they were hanged in a previous life and so on.

For me the information and healing are activated by presence and intention. What I observe over and over again as I work is that:

- Reiki works on the physical, emotional and spiritual levels as each individual requires, requests and is ready to receive. I don't believe anything ever emerges in a session that the client is not ready to deal with, even though the session itself may present as being somewhat traumatic. It is never intended to re-traumatise, only to acknowledge the trauma that took place and then release it from the client's energy field, allowing a return to optimal health and functioning.
- It is an holistic treatment promoting the body's regenerative self healing ability.
- It is concerned with healing causes rather than curing symptoms. This to me represents a key differentiator between ancient healing, which seeks to heal the initial wound or the root cause and scientific, drug based approaches, which frequently aim to cure symptoms. For instance, at least in the UK, anti-depressants are frequently given out to patients without also giving them appropriate therapy to deal with the underlying cause of their depression. Many patients are given drugs or surgery without addressing the bad diet, addictions, lack of exercise or stress that have led to the need for the medical attention and intervention. So long as the symptoms are dealt with, the medical system considers the patient to be 'cured'.
- Intention is key. So for instance when working with the physical body, I ask the Reiki energy to heal each and every cell, to allow each and every cell to work optimally, if that is possible. If there are cells that cannot be healed, such as tumours or scar tissue, I ask for them to be dissolved and released from the body as toxic waste, to be replaced by cells that are working optimally, always in the best interests of the client's Higher Self (more on what I mean by Higher Self will be explained in the chapter on self love).

- I also work in a space of unconditional love. One hugely important lesson from a shamanic healer that I used to visit as a client was never to work with someone if I can't do it from a place of unconditional love, without judgement or imposition of my beliefs. As soon as I work from fear or anger, the energy that I am channelling into the client will not be helpful for them.

So how does Reiki work? As with non-locality and quantum entanglement, there is no really good scientific explanation of how distance healing and energy medicine work, but there is clear evidence that they do.

In the next chapters I look at the growing recognition of the existence and impact of the universal energy field within Western medicine as well as the more traditional Indian and Asian descriptions of the energetic channels. In Chapter 10 I quote some of the studies of alternative and complementary medicine and the evidence for their effectiveness, which is turning from a molehill into a mountain.

It seems highly likely that the full explanation of 'how', when it does emerge, will be a greater understanding of how information is communicated and transformed from the multi-dimensional, microscopic realm of quantum physics to the macroscopic realm of our physical bodies and minds.

Chapter 8:

The Connection between Eastern Energy Terminology and the Endocrine System

'We are not physical machines that have learned how to think.
Perhaps it's the other way around: We are thoughts (and
impulses, consciousness, feelings, emotions, desires and dreams)
that have learned how to create physical bodies; that which we
call our physical body is perhaps just a place that our memories
call home for the time being.'[58] (Deepak Chopra)

My initial investigations, after realising I am more than my physical body, led me to quantum physics, as already described. However, working with Reiki and meditation also required me to gain an understanding of the energy centres within the body and their relationship to our physiology and emotions.

This gradually led me to the relatively new medical fields of psychoneuroimmunology, which links our thoughts, our nervous system and our immune system; and epigenetics, which highlights the extent to which we can control both our endocrine system and our genetic expression.

---

[58] Chopra, Deepak. 2005. Psychology of the Future: Lessons from Modern Consciousness Research, pp204-5 in *Consciousness and Healing*, edited by Schlitz, Marilyn and Amorok, Tina with Micozzi, Marc S.. St Louis, Missouri, USA: Elsevier

Again these were fields I had absolutely no knowledge of until the last couple of years, but as I gained access to them my resounding question became why isn't this information known to everyone, presented in the media and taught in the biology lessons in schools as a standard part of the curriculum? It is so important for all of us and there is so much knowledge and evidence within the medical research community, yet it remains largely hidden from the public unless we dig around for it.

In this and the next two chapters I investigate the scientific evidence that I discovered is emerging to link meditation, energy medicine and traditional shamanic healing practices with modern physiology, neurology and quantum physics.

First of all it is necessary to understand the terminology used in energy medicine. The underlying life force energy is given different names in different cultures, hence it is known as Ki in Japan, Chi in China, Prana in India, Mana in Polynesia and Orenda in Amerindian tribes. The important thing is that no matter what the label, the descriptions of this energy are remarkably similar whichever culture they come from, at whatever period of history. So how does it work?

Three of the most important features of the life force energy perceived and worked with by healers, shamans and meditators around the world, are the **energy sheaths** that surround the physical body, the **nadis** or energy channels within the physical body and the **chakras** or energy centres at specific points within and above the body which appear to transmit energy from the physical realm to the transpersonal. These are explained in greater detail below, along with their perceived links to the endocrine system.

Energy Sheaths

For at least three thousand years the holy books of India, the Upanishads, have been talking of five energy 'sheaths' (kosha) surrounding the body, representing progressively higher levels of vibration.

These layers are:

- The physical sheath, including all physical parts of the body that require food and oxygen for survival.
- The energetic sheath, alternatively called the astral body, the etheric double, the subtle body, the vital sheath or the pranic sheath. It stands specifically for the field of energy that penetrates and surrounds the physical body. It is the medium of exchange in the psychophysiological system. Prana enters at the time of conception and leaves at the time of death of the physical body.
- The mental sheath, which incorporates the sensory motor mind, processing the input from the five senses to form perceptions.
- The intellectual sheath, alternatively called the intelligence sheath, relating to mental functions such as discernment and cognition in states of mystical awareness. This is the organ of philosophical thought, metaphysical intuition and the seat of the human will.
- The blissful sheath, accessible only through ecstatic states or in deep sleep, giving experiences of absolute peace, love and joy.

Beyond these layers and yet forming their very essence is the Soul, also known as the High Self, the Permanent Self, the Spirit or Purusha, which survives after physical death and is part of the all pervading Supreme Spirit, known in the Indian metaphysical literature as Atman. The Atman can travel through space and time, can be launched from one dimension of existence into another and can take up residence time after time in different human bodies to experience the realm of matter and thereby further its development or evolution.

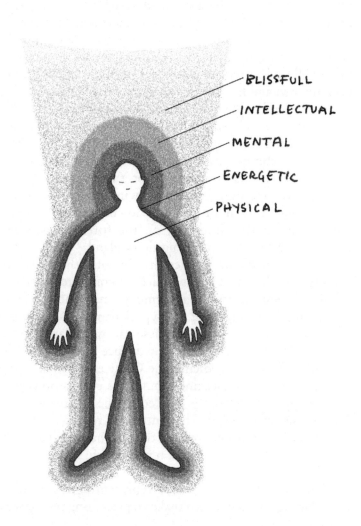

BLISSFULL

INTELLECTUAL

MENTAL

ENERGETIC

PHYSICAL

Nadis

The Nadis are the system of energy channels superimposed on the physical body. All the Nadis originate in the perineum and there are then three universally recognised principle pathways. The central pathway (Sushumna-Nadi) runs along the spine from the root chakra in the perineum to the crown chakra at the top of the head. It is the trajectory of the ascending kundalini energy[59], the awakened serpent power, leading to liberation in the Atman. On the physical level it is the central nervous system, on the energetic level it is the location of the energy centres, the chakras. It carries spiritual energy and is often believed to remain closed off until the other Nadis have been opened and harmonised through yogic practice.

To the left lies the Ida-Nadi, which is symbolised by the cool moon. It is associated with the Goddess and represents the feminine or Yin energy. To the right lies the Pingala-Nadi, which is symbolised by the hot sun. It is associated with the God and represents the masculine or Yang energy.

These Ida and Pingala pathways wind around the Sushumna, intersecting at each of the five lower energy centres and terminating at the third eye, on the forehead between the eyebrows and in front of the pituitary gland.

Chinese medicine teaches that in total there are around seventy-two thousand Nadis, which are connected to the brain's limbic system, controlling memory and emotion and co-ordinating the functions of the hypothalamus and the pituitary.

Its interesting to note that these pathways carrying our life force energy have been represented since ancient times by the symbol of Western medicine, the Caduceus, which represents the entwined Nadis twisting around the chakra power centres and the input of Prana represented by the wings located at the base of the brain chakra. The central rod represents the cosmic fire, the central nervous system, the Shushumna. The entwined snakes of the left and the right represent life and consciousness (the feminine and the masculine). The Caduceus also symbolises the four elements, with the rod representing earth, the wings representing air and the two snakes representing respectively fire and water.

---

[59] Kundalini is a Sanskrit word meaning coiled up, like a snake or a spring. It is traditionally symbolised as a sleeping serpent coiled at the base of the human spine, with the potential to rise through the chakras to the crown allowing the bio-energy to rise and assist on the path to transformation and enlightenment.

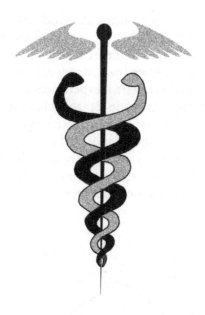

The entwined snakes appear in many mythologies, particularly those of the indigenous people of Australia and Central and Southern America. Their modern relationship to the entwined double helix of DNA was investigated extensively by Dr. Jeremy Narby in *The Cosmic Serpent*,[60] referred to in detail in Chapter 12.

Chakra

As well as working with the sheaths surrounding the physical body, and the channels running through the body, energy medicine for millennia has worked with particular energy centres called chakras. There are seven chakras located within the body, plus one below the feet and one above the crown. The one below the feet is an earth or grounding chakra. It is black and represents our connection with the planet. The one above the crown is a spiritual chakra connecting with the transpersonal.

---

[60] Narby, Jeremy. 1999. *The Cosmic Serpent, DNA and the Origins of Knowledge.* New York, NY, USA: Jeremy P. Tarcher/Putnam

It is clear in colour, representing the God or Goddess within.

There are now literally hundreds of books listing what energy healers associate with each of these chakras. The information I have given here is partially drawn from *Hands of Light*[61] and *Meditation as Medicine*,[62] as well as my own experiences with clients.

What is crucial to connect the chakras with Western medicine and an explanation of how energy healing works, is their linkage with the major glands of the endocrine system, each of which secretes hormones directly into the bloodstream to regulate the body's functions, including metabolism, growth and development, tissue function and mood.

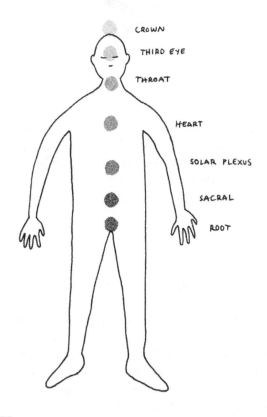

[61] Brennan, Barbara Ann. 1988. *Hands of Light*. USA and Canada: Bantam Books
[62] Singh Khalsa, M.D., Dharma and Stauth, Cameron 2001 *Meditation as Medicine*. New York, NY, USA: Fireside

The major features of each chakra are shown in the table below and more details about the organs, ailments and emotions associated with the first six chakras are in the appendix to this chapter.

Chakra	Name	Colour	Element	Endocrine Gland	Nervous Plexus
First	Base or root	Red	Earth	Gonads (testes and ovaries)	Coccygeal
Second	Sacral	Orange	Water	Adrenals and gonads	Sacral
Third	Solar Plexus	Yellow	Fire	Adrenals and pancreas	Solar
Fourth	Heart	Green/Rose	Air	Thymus	Cardiac/pulmonary
Fifth	Throat	Blue	Ether	Thyroid and para-thyroid	Laryngeal
Sixth	Third Eye	Indigo	Vibration	Pituitary	Brain
Seventh	Crown	Violet/White	Spiritual Vibration	Pineal	Brain

Within the body of this chapter I will only talk in more detail about the seventh chakra, located at the crown of the head, as it appears to provide the link between our physical bodies and altered states of consciousness, hence connection with the universal energy field.

Physically, the crown chakra is associated with the brain and the entire nervous system, as well as the sense of empathy. Physical ailments of the seventh chakra include diseases of the nervous system such as depression, paralysis and multiple sclerosis and problems with the hair and nails.

Most importantly it is associated with the pineal gland, the master gland of the endocrine system, situated within the deep recesses of the central nervous system. It is known that the pineal gland produces the hormone melatonin, which controls our sleep pattern and which is also a powerful antioxidant and free-radical scavenger, so any deterioration of the pineal gland contributes to an overall decrease in health. It can also produce the hallucinogen dimethyltryptamine (DMT), a beta-carboline synthesised from melatonin, as well as at least two other hallucinogenic beta-carbolinese. DMT is exactly the hallucinogenic substance contained in the chacruna leaves which are used along with the monoamine oxidase inhibitor Banisteriopsis Caapi in the brew known as ayahuasca that the Amazonian shamans ingest exogenously, which they claim allows them to communicate with the plant world – more of which in Chapter 12.

Unfortunately, since 1971 DMT has been on the controlled substances list, along with synthetic compounds such as heroin and LSD. This means that scientific studies on its effects are rare. However, more information can be found in *DMT: The Spirit Molecule*, [63] by Dr. Rick Strassman. In 1990, when he was Associate Professor of Psychiatry at New Mexico University's School of Medicine, he succeeded in getting funding for a five year long study of DMT, where the subjects were all experienced hallucinogen users who chose to participate in the research. He found substantial evidence that the pineal gland is the source of DMT production and assimilation. It is produced endogenously in specific circumstances, including during birth, death, near-death experiences, and other 'mystical' states, including what meditators would call our access to the superconscious.

Emotionally, the crown is regarded as being the centre of our cosmic consciousness and spirituality and it represents the soul – the part of us that continues lifetime after lifetime. At this level of the superconscious we are all connected in what is known by various names, including the Oneness or the Atman.

---

[63] Strassman, M.D., Rick. 2001. *DMT: The Spirit Molecule – A Doctor's Revolutionary Research into the Biology of Near-Death and Mystical Experiences.* Rochester, Vermont, USA: Park Street Press

Ill health and the endocrine system

The endocrine system produces the hormones which control many body functions and organs, as well as behaviour. Almost inevitably, ill health results when hormone concentrations are either too high or too low. The amount of any hormone that is released is dependent on the interaction of the hypothalamus section of the brain and the pituitary gland. The secretion of hypothalamic hormones is dependent on a wide range of stimuli, including nervous, metabolic, physical and hormonal. This last factor leads to one of the major distinguishing features of the endocrine system: the prevalence of feedback loops, both positive and negative, which are used extensively to regulate the secretion of hormones in the hypothalamic-pituitary axis.

For instance thyrotrophic-releasing hormone (TRH) is released by the hypothalamus and stimulates the production of thyroid stimulating hormone (TSH) in the pituitary. This in turn stimulates the thyroid gland which releases thyoxine and tri-iodothyronine. If the levels of these two chemicals are low, the hypothalamus increases its production of TRH to stimulate the production of more TSH in the pituitary. If the levels of thyoxine and tri-iodothyronine are high, the hypothalamus reduces the secretion of TRH. So it is a two way flow of information between the glands, the pituitary and the hypothalamus.

Unfortunately, the functions of the hypothalamus, the pineal gland and the endocrine are amongst the first to wear out as we age, leading to a wide variety of stresses, illnesses and disease – unless we can take action to keep them healthy, which is one of the major objectives of both meditation and energy work with the chakras.

Uses in Reiki and other energy healing

It is important for energy healers to be aware of the different features of all the chakras and their interaction with different organs and emotions, as these give good signposts to the underlying cause of energetic blockages felt at different parts of the body.

My job when I am working with a client is to open myself to connection with their energy field, sensing the subtle vibrations throughout their body and places where those vibrations are stuck, or feel heavy or dark. Connecting into their system and acknowledging the underlying traumas and pain that are locked into their tissues and their energy fields allows change and release, partially because the work encourages the client's endocrine system to release different hormones as described in the next chapter, transforming the body from a place of disease to health.

Appendix to Chapter 6

The first chakra at the base of the spine is physically associated with elimination, the lymph system, the prostate gland, the bladder and the colon. It is also connected with smell, hence is associated with the nose. In connection with the endocrine system it is associated with the gonads which orchestrate our sexual and reproductive functions.

Physical ailments include constipation, lower back pain, haemorrhoids, sciatica, knee problems, addictive sex behaviour, depression, colorectal cancer, irritable bowel syndrome, colitis and Crohn's disease.

Emotionally, the root is the place of birth and rebirth, and it is associated with those parts of the consciousness concerned with ego, security, survival and trust. These frequently manifest as concerns about money, home or job, not feeling at home, not being grounded, or difficulty being present here and now, wanting to live or die.

The root chakra also stores information about each person's relationship with their mother, which sets the pattern for relationship with everything that represents security. Blockages in the root chakra may derive from a feeling of separation from mother, not being loved or nourished by her. This separation leads to viewing the world from a position of insecurity or fear.

The second chakra behind the lower abdomen is physically associated with reproduction and the senses of taste and appetite. It is linked to the uterus, spleen, kidneys, bladder and tongue. In connection with the endocrine system it is linked again to the gonads and also to the adrenals, which sit below the rib cage, capping each kidney. The adrenals produce the hormones which control such functions as body fluids, the breakdown of protein, the amount of blood glucose, total body fat, the production of anti-bodies to deal with infection and inflammation, and the secretion of adrenalin, which triggers the fight or flight response. They also produce sex hormones controlling sexual development and maturity, and ovulation.

Physical ailments of the second chakra include lower back pain, fertility problems, fibroids, cystitis, kidney problems and muscle cramps or spasms.

Emotionally, the second chakra is related to motivation, with what turns us on emotionally, sexual choosing and creativity, which may manifest themselves as tensions about food, worries about having children, relationships or suppression of emotion. It's also associated with guilt and anxiety about money and low self-esteem. Imbalance may be manifested as isolation if the chakra's energy is too weak, and as lust if the energy is too strong. It is the centre of self-knowledge and is home to the self you need to love. It is about connecting deeply with the spirit that moves through you.

The third chakra behind the naval is physically associated with the liver, kidneys, gall bladder, large intestine, middle back, muscular system or skin as a system and the sense of sight. It controls growth and balance. In connection with the endocrine system it is again associated with the adrenals and also with the pancreas which secretes insulin and glucagon, helping to regulate blood sugar levels.

Physical ailments include digestive problems, alcoholism, hepatitis, gallstones, food issues (anorexia, allergies, diabetes etc), and ulcers.

Emotionally, the solar plexus is associated with issues of power and judgement, and other emotions based on fear, anxiety, insecurity, jealousy, anger, control and freedom. These are ego issues and tension in the third chakra can also be a sign of conflict between one's ego or personality and one's Higher Self. A person with a strong third chakra feels perpetually confident, almost with an ethereal umbilical cord, connecting the person to the power of the universe. To this person, the world is a nurturing entity, not the difficult world that is experienced by a person with a weak third chakra.

The solar plexus is the force behind our will – our ability to act consciously, to make decisions and then follow them through knowing that we will achieve success.

The fourth chakra behind the heart is associated with the heart itself, blood pressure, the lungs, bronchial tubes, upper back, arms and hands and the sense of touch.

In connection with the endocrine system it is associated with the thymus, the most important single gland of the immune system. Its function is to transform lymphocytes (white blood cells developed in the bone marrow) into T-cells (cells developed in the thymus). These cells are then transported to various lymph glands, where they play an important part in fighting infections and disease.

Physical ailments include breast cancer, heart disease and problems with the immune system such as HIV/AIDS.

Emotionally, the heart is the place of love, the soul, inner guidance, and the 'higher emotions' based on unconditional love, empathy, compassion and friendship. When energy is blocked in the heart chakra the balance between giving and receiving can become distorted. Often, how we feel about being touched will help identify emotional problems in the heart chakra. Breathing problems may reflect difficulty in making decisions about letting love in and out and opening the heart chakra is often about a process of self-acceptance, replacing self-judgement with self-love.

The fifth chakra located in the throat, is associated with the ears, nose, throat and also the arms and hands, the aspects of expressing and receiving as well as the sense of hearing. In connection with the endocrine system it is associated with the thyroid and parathyroid glands, which produce the hormones which control the general metabolic rate, the heartbeat, the blood pressure, mental activity, fertility and growth, as well as maintaining the correct level of calcium in the plasma and the kidneys.

Physical ailments of the fifth chakra include eating disorders such as anorexia, bulimia and constant dieting, as well as problems of metabolism controlled by the thyroid gland.

Psychological issues about how much space we take up in the world often cause obsessions with weight.

Emotionally it is associated with communication and expression, truth, the true expression of the soul and creativity and willpower. It is linked to our beliefs concerning the potential for the manifestation of our goals. It is associated with the process of listening to intuition and the state of consciousness we experience when we flow with that process – often referred to as abundance, or grace. Thus tension in these areas can represent holding back from achieving goals, resistance to expressing what is wanted or felt.

Psychic ability and communion with those from other realms resonates at the throat centre. We learn to connect with our spirit guides, ancestors, angels and helpers through the throat chakra and the ether element.

The sixth chakra, between the eyebrows, is associated with the hypothalamus, brain, eyes and face and the sense of vision. It is also associated with all the inner senses that correspond to each of the outer physical senses, such as clairvoyance, clairaudience, etc.

In terms of the endocrine system it is associated with the pituitary gland, which is approximately the size of a pea and is located near the middle of the brain, along with the other limbic structures. The pituitary gland works in a feedback loop with all the other endocrine glands by relaying 'hormone orders' between the hypothalamus and the amygdala, the emotional centre of the brain, and the endocrine glands, instructing them to produce more of the chemicals needed to maintain proper balance in the body.

Physical ailments include mental illness, cognitive disorders and problems of physical growth as our biological structure changes in accordance with and as the effect of our perceptions. Learning difficulties, brain tumours, blindness, deafness, pain and insomnia can originate here.

Emotionally, the sixth chakra is the centre of our psychic perception, consciousness, awareness, intuition and soul knowledge. From here we can visualise our destiny and make it our reality.

Chapter 9:
Dr. Larry Dossey's Eras of Healing

'Memories are stored not only in the brain, but in a psychosomatic network extending into the body, particularly in the ubiquitous receptors between nerves and bundles of cell bodies called ganglia, which are distributed not just in and near the spinal cord, but all the way out along pathways to internal organs and the very surface of the skin. The decision about what becomes a thought rising to consciousness and what remains an undigested thought pattern buried at a deeper level in the body is mediated by the receptors.' [64] (Candace Pert)

Having described the terminology of energy medicine and the connections between the chakras and the endocrine system in the previous chapter, I would like to move on to the medical evidence linking our physical bodies and brains/neurological systems, which is heavily dependent on the functioning of the endocrine system, before tackling the research studies linking our physical bodies with the non-local mind in Chapter 10.

Dr. Larry Dossey served as a battalion surgeon in Vietnam, where he was decorated for valour. He went on to help establish

---

[64] Pert Ph.D., Candace B. 1999. *Molecules of Emotion, Why You Feel the Way You Feel.* p.143. London, UK: Simon & Schuster

the Dallas Diagnostic Association and was Chief of Staff of Medical City Dallas Hospital in 1982. He lectures at major medical schools and hospitals around the world, focusing on the 'non-local mind', mind unconfined to the brain and body, mind spread infinitely throughout space and time.

He describes three distinct types or 'Eras' of healing methodology[65].

- Era I believes all forms of therapy are physical and the body is regarded as a mechanism that functions according to deterministic principles. This encompasses most of 'modern' medical technology. Mind or consciousness is equated with the functioning of the brain.
- Era II describes the mind-to-body medical approaches that involve the psychosomatic effects of one's consciousness on one's own body, i.e. what you think affects your health. But mind is still seen as a function of brain chemistry and anatomy. These therapies include psychosomatic medicine, biofeedback, hypnosis, meditation etc.
- In Era III medicine, mind is seen as unconfined by either space or time: it is boundless and unlimited. It is recognised that our non-local mind may affect healing both within and between people. Noncontact healing modalities between people in each others' presence, as well as between people distant from each other, become possible with non-local mind.

Reiki and other energy healing practices have features of both Era II and Era III medicine, so let's look first at the growing science of Era II healing.

Psychoneuroimmunology and Era II healing

Dr. Candace Pert has been one of the pioneers of the field of psychoneuroimmunology (PNI) since 1970. PNI is the area of

---

[65] http://www.dossey.com/larry/QnA.html

medical research which connects our thoughts (psyche), our nervous system (neurology) and our immune system to prove that what we think affects our health. Initially she was ostracised for her insights, but she has now been re-embraced by the establishment medical community. She has served as Chief of the Section on Brain Biochemistry in the Clinical Neuroscience Branch of the National Institute of Mental Health (NIMH), held a Research Professorship in the Department of Physiology and Biophysics at Georgetown University School of Medicine in Washington, DC and is currently the Scientific Director of RAPID Laboratories, Inc. This section relies very heavily on her book, *Molecules of Emotion*[66], to which I am heavily indebted.

In a nutshell, PNI has demonstrated that *'the three classically separated areas of neuroscience, endocrinology, and immunology, with their various organs – the brain; the glands; and the spleen, bone marrow, and lymph nodes – are actually joined to each other in a multidirectional network of communication, linked by information carriers known as neuropeptides.'*[67]

Some of the key components in this linkage are the massive, complex molecules known as receptors, which are found floating on the surface of cells in the body and brain. A typical nerve cell may have millions of receptors on its surface. These receptors cluster in the cellular membrane waiting for the right chemical keys to arrive through the extracellular fluid and mount them by fitting into their keyholes, a process known as binding.

The chemical key that docks onto the receptor is called a ligand. Ligands include hormones, neurotransmitters and peptides. As Pert describes it *'Ligand is the term used for any natural or manmade substance that binds selectively to its own specific receptor on the surface of a cell... The ligand bumping on is what we call the binding and in the process, the ligand transfers a message via its molecular properties to the receptor...*

'The receptor, having received a message, transmits it from the surface of the cell deep into the cell's interior, where the

---

[66] Pert Ph.D., Candace B. 1999. *Molecules of Emotion, Why You Feel the Way You Feel.* London, U.K.: Simon & Schuster

[67] Pert Ph.D., Candace B. 1999. *Molecules of Emotion, Why You Feel the Way You Feel.* p.184 London, U.K.: Simon & Schuster

message can change the state of the cell dramatically. A chain reaction of biochemical events is initiated... and, directed by the message of the ligand, begin any number of activities – manufacturing new proteins, making decisions about cell division, opening or closing ion channels, adding or subtracting energetic chemical groups like the phosphates – to name just a few. In short, the life of the cell, what it is up to at any moment, is determined by which receptors are on its surface, and whether those receptors are occupied by ligands or not.'[68]

The discovery that Pert and her colleagues made, which was shocking and revolutionary at the time, forty years ago, was that ligands and receptors are not just in the nervous system and the brain as previously thought, attached to synapses to pass signals, but are distributed throughout the body. And the largest portion of information held in the body is '*kept in order not by the synaptic connections of brain cells but by the specificity of the receptors – in other words, by the ability of the receptor to bind with only one kind of ligand... Counter to the collective wisdom of the neuropharmacologists and neuroscientists, less than 2 percent of neuronal communication actually occurs at the synapse.*'[69]

The neuropeptide ligands and other informational substances which travel throughout the body are the bio-chemicals which lead to the emotions we feel such as hunger, anger, pain, relaxation, sexual drive. Over two hundred peptides have been mapped to different emotions, which appear to be associated with different vibrational rates of the receptor molecules, which open and close with a rhythmic, pumping action, so '*their distribution in the body's nerves has all kinds of significance... The body is the unconscious mind! Repressed traumas caused by overwhelming emotion can be stored in a body part, thereafter affecting our ability to feel that part or even move it.*'[70] in the Nervous System

[68] Pert Ph.D., Candace B. 1999. *Molecules of Emotion, Why You Feel the Way You Feel.* p.24 London, U.K.: Simon & Schuster
[69] Pert Ph.D., Candace B. 1999. *Molecules of Emotion, Why You Feel the Way You Feel.* p.139 London, U.K.: Simon & Schuster
[70] Pert Ph.D., Candace B. 1999. *Molecules of Emotion, Why You Feel the Way You Feel.* p.141 London, U.K.: Simon & Schuster

Pert continues that it has also been proved, '*that biochemical change wrought at the receptor level is the molecular basis of memory. When a receptor is flooded with a ligand, it changes the cell membrane in such a way that the probability of an electrical impulse travelling across the membrane where the receptor resides is facilitated or inhibited, thereafter affecting the choice of neuronal circuitry that will be used.*'[71]

The result is that '*Emotional states or moods are produced by the various neuropeptide ligands, and what we experience as an emotion or a feeling is also a mechanism for activating a particular neuronal circuit – simultaneously throughout the brain and body – which generates a behaviour involving the whole creature, with all the necessary physiological changes that behaviour would require.*'[72]

In other words, what we think consciously and what we experience emotionally are both to some extent the result of the physiological behaviour of the endocrine system and the hormones it releases throughout the system. At the same time the endocrine system is responsible for the health (ease) or sickness (dis-ease) of each and every cell in our bodies. And each and every tissue in our bodies holds memories of key incidents as a result of the ligands that were released and bound to the receptors on those tissues when the incident occurred.

So for instance, the simple act of breathing in different ways (for example during a rebirthing or yoga session) or receiving bodywork, can change the type and quantity of peptide ligands produced by the brain stem, leading to a change in physical health.

This occurs because the lungs are filled with a very high concentration of peptides and communicate with the periaqueductal grey area (PAG) located in the aqueduct that connects the third and fourth ventricles in the midbrain via the peptides carried in the cerebrospinal fluid. By breathing deeply,

[71] Pert Ph.D., Candace B. 1999. *Molecules of Emotion, Why You Feel the Way You Feel.* p.143. London, U.K.: Simon & Schuster
[72] Pert Ph.D., Candace B. 1999. *Molecules of Emotion, Why You Feel the Way You Feel.* p.145 London, U.K.: Simon & Schuster

or rapidly, or by holding your breath, you can change the profile of pulmonary peptides that communicate with your PAG. The PAG is the site of the body's largest supply of opiate receptors and the linkage between the opiate receptors and the pulmonary peptides helps determine the level of pain, anger and fear a person is feeling. Thus as you change the profile of pulmonary peptides reaching the PAG through changing the way you breathe, you can change how you feel, providing self-control over pain, anger and fear.

Similarly, meditation, breathwork and bodywork can be used to release neuropeptide ligands throughout the body. As they begin to circulate, these ligands can allow people to feel emotions that have been shut down for many years and make new choices about their lives.

The frontal cortex, the forebrain, is the location for all the higher cognitive functions, such as planning for the future, making decisions, and formulating intentions to change. It needs adequate nourishment which is carried as glucose by the blood. Only when there is enough blood flow to bring plentiful supplies of glucose to the brain are the neurones and glial cells able to carry on their functions fully. This blood flow in turn is closely regulated by neuropeptides which signal receptors on blood vessels to constrict or dilate.

If we block our emotions through denial or repression, then the flow of blood can become chronically constricted, depriving the frontal cortex of proper nourishment. This leaves us limited in awareness and the ability to make choices. As a result we can become stuck and unable to respond freshly to the world around us, repeating old patterns of behaviour and with feelings that are responses to an outdated knowledge base. As the emotions are brought up and acknowledged, different neuropeptide ligands start to flow, signalling the receptors to behave differently and allowing the blood flow to increase. This improves our ability to make choices which then enhance the positive endocrine feedback system.

Stress is another well known major inhibitor of neuropeptide flow which results in a suppression of the active functioning of the immune system thereby upsetting the body's normal healing response.

By learning to unblock past repressed experiences and emotions, memories which are stored in the very receptors of your cells, you can release yourself from these blocked traumas and conditioning as well as the associated physical responses, returning the body and the emotions to health. We can also learn techniques to relax and offset the impact of stress on our system, enhancing the ability of our immune systems to fend off any viruses or diseases that enter from our environment.

Once again I have had many personal experiences of the power and validity of this approach and the interdependency between our physical health and our mental belief systems.

One particular example derived from my repressed sexuality. My partner Sean enjoyed sex enormously without shame or guilt and quite reasonably expected me to do the same. I tried to please him, doing what to most consenting adults would be perfectly normal, but which to me, in my core energy field and limiting belief system was still 'sinful'. About five months after we became lovers I developed chronic cystitis, which I ignored, and which developed into pyelonephritis – a severe kidney infection, which had me hospitalised for the first time in my adult life, apart from during childbirth.

I recovered after five days hooked up to anti-biotics and drips, but realised that the whole infection had come along because of the resistance to sex still held in my tissue memory. This was unconsciously held as tension in my vagina and cervix, leading to cystitis on penetration. What we believe affects our health. This lesson led me to much further work learning first to accept and then to love and honour my sexuality. That particular aspect of my journey is described in Chapter 13.

Since then I have worked with a number of women with chronic cystitis and urinary tract infections. Frequently they have suffered from incest or abusive sex and are continuing to feel shame and guilt, sometimes decades later, which is stored as tension in their tissue memory, which results in pain when having sex, leading naturally to a reluctance to engage in a healthy, active, joyful sex life.

As I work with them to revisit the initial traumas and then acknowledge that the accompanying limiting beliefs are no longer necessary or serve them, they are able to release their self-hatred and anger and move into a place of honouring their femininity and their sexual organs. Almost inevitably this changes the type of men they attract into their lives and the quality of their relationships going forward.

Epigenetics

Identifying the inter-connectedness between our physiology and our emotions was the first step for the medical community in acknowledging that thoughts and feelings can make us physically ill, or alternatively can heal us – what until then had been thought of as 'psychosomatic' in a very negative, deprecating way. A second step towards recognising that we hold the keys to our own health is the rapidly growing field of epigenetics which highlights the extent to which we are in charge of the expression of our genetic inheritance.

With the discovery of deoxyribonucleic acid (DNA) it became fashionable to believe that our health is genetically determined, according to the gene sequences encoded in our DNA, passed down to us from our parents.

Epigenetics is the science of how environmental signals select, modify and regulate gene activity leading to heritable changes in gene function that occur **without** a change in the DNA sequence.

How is such a thing possible? Genes of course do exist in our DNA, but what matters to our health is whether they are turned on or off. Epigenetics studies the signals that turn genes on and off. Some of those signals are chemical, others are electromagnetic. Some come from the environment inside the body, while others are our body's response to signals from the environment that surrounds our body.

Within our bodies, DNA forms the core of every chromosome. Protein molecules on either side of the cell membrane cover the DNA like a sleeve. When genes are covered, their information cannot be read. To allow genes to be uncovered and activated, you need a signal to tell the protein covering to detach from the DNA's double helix.

Dawson Church is the founder of the Soul Medicine

97

Institute[73], a non-profit institution dedicated to education and research into science based medical interventions which use consciousness and energy as primary modalities.

In *Genie in your Genes* he provides a simplified explanation of how this environmental signalling works. *'There are protein molecules on either side of the cell membrane. The proteins on the external surfaces of the cell are receptive to external forces, including the biochemical changes in the body produced by different kinds of thought and emotion. These external receptors in turn affect the internal proteins, altering their molecular angles. The two sets of receptors function like a lattice work that can expand or contract. The degree of expansion determines the size and shape of the molecules – so called 'effector proteins' – that can pass through the lattice. Together the 'receptor-effector complex' acts as a molecular switch, accepting signals from the cell's environment that trigger the unwrapping of the protein sleeve around DNA.'*[74]

The conclusion is that causality runs from environmental signals to the presence or absence of protein sleeves, to covering or uncovering of the DNA to whether the gene is switched on or not. So whether or not a 'genetic trait' is activated or not depends on a host of environmental factors, many of which are within our control.

Hence, *'Two individuals might have an identical genetic sequence for a particular disease encoded in their cells. The beliefs of the one individual provide the signals that unwrap the protein covering and allow the gene to be activated; the beliefs of the other individual do not.'*[75] If the gene was connected with a medical condition, in the first case the individual would get the disease, in the second case they would not.

Thus it is our emotional environment and our conditioned belief systems as well as the toxicity or health of the food that

---

[73] http://www.soulmedicineinstitute.org/
[74] Church Ph.D., Dawson. 2007. *The Genie in Your Genes, Epigenetic Medicine and the New Biology of Intention.* p.169 Llandeilo, U.K.: Cygnus Books
[75] Church Ph.D., Dawson. 2007. *The Genie in Your Genes, Epigenetic Medicine and the New Biology of Intention.* p.169 Llandeilo, U.K.: Cygnus Books

we eat and the ecological systems that we are surrounded by that determine our health. As Church put it, *'Memory, learning, stress and healing are all affected by classes of genes that are turned on or off in temporal cycles that range from one second to many hours. The environment that activates genes includes both the inner environment – the emotional, biochemical, mental, energetic and spiritual landscape of the individual – and the outer environment. The outer environment includes the social network and ecological systems in which the individual lives. Food, toxins, social rituals and sexual cues are examples of outer environmental influences that affect gene expression. Researchers estimate that approximately 90% of all genes are engaged... in cooperation with signals from the environment.'*[76]

In *The Biology of Belief* Lipton reports that many different studies have found epigenetic mechanisms to be a factor in a variety of diseases, including cancer, cardiovascular disease and diabetes. *'The malignancies in a significant number of cancer patients are derived from environmentally induced epigenetic alterations and not defective genes. Recently eminent scientist and physician Dean Ornish revealed that by just changing diet and lifestyle for 90 days, prostate cancer patients switched the activity of over 500 genes. Many of their gene changes inhibited biological processes critical in the formation of their tumours.'*[77,78]

The other dramatic finding has been that not only can we impact our own genes, we can also change the expression of the genes we pass on to our children without changing the genes themselves.

Church describes in some detail[79] the experiments carried out at McGill University in Montreal, Canada, to validate this

---

[76] Church Ph.D., Dawson. 2007. *The Genie in Your Genes, Epigenetic Medicine and the New Biology of Intention.* p.33. Llandeilo, U.K.: Cygnus Books
[77] Lipton Ph.D., Bruce H. 2005. *The Biology of Belief, Unleashing the Power of Consciousness, Matter & Miracles.* p.42 Carlsbad, CA, USA: Hay House, Inc.
[78] Ornish, Dean, Magbanua, M.J. et al. 2008. *Changes in prostate gene expression in men undergoing an intensive nutrition and lifestyle intervention.* Proceedings of the National Academy of Sciences. 105: 8369-8374
[79] Church Ph.D., Dawson. 2007. *The Genie in Your Genes, Epigenetic Medicine and the New Biology of Intention.* p.54 Llandeilo, U.K.: Cygnus Books

proposition. Rats whose mothers nurtured them well had a prevalence of certain genes in the hippocampus that dampened their response to stress and they also showed more acetyl chemicals which make it easier for these stress-dampening genes to express. On the other hand, the rats whose mothers did not spend so much time licking them and grooming them showed anxiety and stress. These rats had more gene suppressing methyl groups in their hippocampi. These bond to the DNA and inhibit the expression of the gene involved in dampening stress. The well-nurtured rats acted in a similar way towards their own offspring as they had been treated, extending the behavioural results to the next generation.

The implication of epigenetics is of course that we have a significant degree of control over our cells, our genetic activation, our overall health and wellbeing, through our lifestyle choices, our dietary choices and where and how we decide to live. We also impact the health and wellbeing of our children by how we treat them, what we feed them, where we choose to live and what we teach them to believe.

The Science of Yoga and Meditation

Meditation is probably the most widely studied Era II medicine and has repeatedly demonstrated the extent of our ability to be co-creators of our own health.

Dr. Dharma Singh Khalsa is President and medical director of the Alzheimer's Prevention Foundation in Tucson, Arizona. He is also a yogi and conducts workshops on brain longevity and Medical Meditation. In *Meditation as Medicine*[80] he describes the chakras as the ethereal components of our physical nerve plexuses, organs and glands. He believes they exchange energy bi-directionally, between the physical and ethereal.

He emphasises that chakras can be impaired as a result of sudden shock, trauma, fear, anxiety and stress. Psychological

---

[80] Singh Khalsa, M.D., Dharma and Stauth, Cameron 2001 *Meditation as Medicine*. New York, NY, USA: Fireside

problems may cause blockages obstructing the flow of energy into or out of the chakras. Such obstruction in the energy flow can result in an erratic endocrine gland functioning, impacting the quantity and quality of peptide production and leading to a consequent imbalance of the hormone activity.

Singh Khalsa reports the conclusions of studies by the US Federal Government's Office of Alternative Medicine on meditation and Dr. Herbert Benson of the Harvard Medical School.

- *'Hundreds of studies have been performed and they indicate the following:*
- *'Meditation creates a unique hypometabolic state in which the metabolism is in a deeper state of rest than during sleep.*
- *'Meditation is the only activity that reduces blood lactate, a marker of stress and anxiety.*
- *'The calming hormones melatonin and serotonin are increased by meditation and the stress hormone cortisol is decreased.*
- *'Meditation has a profound effect upon three key indicators of ageing: hearing ability, blood pressure and vision of close objects.*
- *'Long-term meditators experience 80% less heart disease and 50% less cancer than non-meditators.*
- *'Meditators secrete more of the youth-related hormone DHEA as they age than non-meditators.'*[81]

He reports that those who practice Transcendental Meditation also have a lower biological age (measured by physiological determinants rather than chronological age) than those who do not meditate. For those meditating for more than five years, they were physiologically twelve years younger than non-meditating counterparts.[82]

---

[81] Singh Khalsa, M.D., Dharma and Stauth, Cameron 2001 *Meditation as Medicine.* pp7-8 New York, NY, USA: Fireside
[82] Singh Khalsa, M.D., Dharma and Stauth, Cameron 2001 *Meditation as Medicine.* p.44 New York, NY, USA: Fireside

There are now millions of people in the Western world practising a wide variety of yogas and meditations and there are hundreds of books describing the philosophy and techniques and benefits of these practices, which have been in use in India, China and Japan for several thousand years. Many of the schools of yoga focus on opening the kundalini energy channels from the root to the crown, using breathing techniques known as pranayama to restore balance in the chakras.

But of course the ultimate aim of yoga and meditation is not just physical health. It is the attainment of transcendental gnosis or enlightenment, and the yogic scriptures provide many methods to assist in attaining higher states of consciousness, including visualisation, light, sound (mantra), geometric devices (yantra) and ritual action.

How does this work? Again it seems to go back to the connections between our thoughts, our emotions and the endocrine system, with the act of meditation directly rejuvenating the hypothalamus, the pituitary, and the pineal and other endocrine glands. This allows the pineal to release DMT, the molecule which appears to enhance our receptivity to connecting 'non-locally'. Using the metaphor of the holographic universe, meditation helps us to become like the right kind of light source, vibrating at the right frequencies to read the information embedded within the holographic universe.

Over the years I have worked with and explored a great variety of meditation practices. There is not a 'one size fits all' meditation process! Beginners are often taught 'mindfulness', from the Buddhist tradition, which observes the breath as it flows in and out of the nostrils and notices the thoughts passing through the chattering brain without following them and getting hooked into their story. It is our 'stories' which tends to lead us out of the present moment into either past or future. Much of the purpose is to 'be' rather than to 'do', to be the observer of ourselves and to live in the now.

Singh Khalsa explains, *'When you meditate, your rational thought processes, housed in your cortex, begin a quiet dialogue with your brain's emotional centres, the hippocampus and the amygdala, both of which are in your limbic system. When your cortex and limbic system agree that it is appropriate to relax, they relay the message to the hypothalamus, which connects the brain to the endocrine system. This releases a flood of calming neurotransmitters and hormones, which soothe the entire body.*

'The immune system then secretes its own molecules of information, some of which return to the brain, helping to complete this circuitry of healing. You shift into a relaxed alpha brain wave pattern and your nervous system is dominated by the inhibitory parasympathetic branch. When the parasympathetic nervous system is favoured you send relatively more nerve signals to your organs and glands of immunity, such as your thymus. As this occurs you reach the ideal condition for healing – what the mystics call the sacred space.'[83]

Interestingly, it appears that the ancient Sanskrit mantras which are often chanted to accompany meditation have the very specific physiological action of vibrating the pituitary, thereby altering the secretions of this master gland of the endocrine system. The vibrations arising from these mantras can also stimulate the hypothalamus and the vagus nerve which travels through the neck, services the heart, lungs, intestinal tract and back muscles, and they influence the nadis and chakras by vibrating the upper palate of the mouth which has eighty-four points connected to the body's ethereal energy system.

Personal experience of meditation

Over the years I have engaged in a number of meditation practices, just a few of which I describe below as they brought me particular insights.

In 2010 I sat in silence for twelve days in Chennai, India, participating in a Vipassana meditation course, based on a particular variation of Buddhism. During that process you sit in meditation for about ten and a half hours a day. The five precepts, or rules, for the duration of the course, are to abstain

---

[83] Singh Khalsa, M.D., Dharma and Stauth, Cameron 2001 *Meditation as Medicine.* p.30 New York, NY, USA: Fireside

from killing any being; to abstain from stealing; to abstain from all sexual activity; to abstain from telling lies; to abstain from all intoxicants.

As with mindfulness, the Vipassana practice starts with observing the breath coming in and out through the nostrils, before taking your awareness gradually through your whole body, until you acknowledge how each part of your body is feeling at that precise moment, knowing that whatever pain and suffering it is feeling 'this too will pass'. It is a practice based on non-attachment, non-desire and control of the body.

Wake up time is 4.00am, breakfast is at 6.30am, lunch is at 11.30am and then you get a cup of tea and a piece of fruit at 4.30pm. That's it.

For me that particular practice simply didn't work. I was bored, agitated, pissed off, in pain from sitting cross-legged for so long and hungry. I can confess that I spent the last two days focusing on the beer, pizza and chocolate brownie I was going to eat as soon as I was released from the programme, in complete contradiction to its intention of teaching participants to let go of attachment and desire. I was even more pissed off when I weighed myself at a massage centre two days after the course finished and discovered I had gained weight during it despite the lack of food! Sitting for ten and half hours a day doesn't burn a lot of calories I guess.

But what it did make me think about and acknowledge is that I don't want to live on a flat line of equanimity. I believe part of the human condition is to experience the highs and the lows. I also know that for me personally and for clients I have worked with, the suffering and the difficult times, although painful as we experience them, sometimes provide some of the greatest teachings, lessons and gifts in our lives. I do accept that we should not become attached to the highs, so I do accept the philosophy of non-attachment, but that doesn't mean we can't experience, appreciate and benefit from both highs and lows.

However, for millions of people around the world including certain individuals during the course that I participated in, Vipassana does work. It changes people's lives and leads them into a new understanding of their body and its attachments and the way we impose suffering on ourselves. Once more you can only decide if it's the right path for you by experiencing it. Even if it's not right, the experience will bring lessons, as it undoubtedly did for me. So yes, I am glad I participated and completed the programme, even if I won't choose to do it again.

I have also participated in two ten day long tantric meditation courses at Osho Nisarga, just outside Dharamsala, Northern India, working through the one hundred and twelve meditations presented in Osho's *Book of Secrets*,[84] under the supervision of Ma Ananda Sarita, a truly amazing teacher with a continuous offering of courses around the world and some fantastic books on the traditions of tantra and sacred sexuality.[85] Osho never intended people to practice all his one hundred and twelve suggested meditation techniques, but rather he presented them as options, so that people could test them all out and discover which two or three work best for them. They cover a wide range of styles, alone and in couples, indoors and in nature.

For me some were easy, some were near impossible, some were painful, some led to incredible insights. Today there is one in particular that I continue to use in my personal meditation practice and another that I frequently recommend to clients, even if I don't call it a meditation.

The last technique I would like to mention here is mantra based meditation. I worked with this particular technique within the Lucis Trust system for six months.[86] The mantras are short phrases which are repeated and focused on over and over again, so that rather than emptying the mind of thoughts, the intention is to focus the mind on specific, spiritually uplifting and challenging concepts. For me this is a powerful way of disengaging the chattering brain and staying in the present moment, with a particular focus of attention. I find it can be a very powerful way of releasing limiting beliefs and it can be used in conjunction with any affirmation or soul contract you want to focus on and manifest within your life.

---

[84] Osho. 1974. *The Book of Secrets.* New York NY, USA: Osho International Foundation
[85] http://www.ananda-sarita.com/links/
[86] http://www.lucistrust.org/

Conclusions of Era II medicine

Overall, it is only experience that can demonstrate which Era II healing techniques prove most helpful to you personally, from the wide variety of meditation techniques and energy healing methods that are available today. Which ones are most helpful may also change over time as you evolve and progress with your practices. There are many options out there, many roads to enlightenment, no one-size-fits-all prescription.

Deepak Chopra is a well known Indian-born, American doctor, public speaker and writer. He began his medical career as an endocrinologist before shifting his research and work to spirituality, Ayurveda[87] and mind-body medicine. He now runs his own medical centre in California. In a chapter within *Consciousness and Healing*, titled *Timeless Mind, Ageless Body*, he writes, *'We are discovering that our body is actually the objective experience of consciousness, just as our mind is the subjective experience of consciousness. But they're both inseparably one.*

'You and I are neither the body nor the mind; we are the creator of both, which is pure consciousness. It's difficult sometimes to express this in words, but this has been, in fact, the wisdom of almost every spiritual tradition in the world.' [88] (Deepak Chopra)

Some of my own healing work falls into Era II medicine, doing bodywork with the client to access and release deeply held limiting beliefs, memories, trauma and repressed emotions that are stored in the body, the tissues and the deep unconscious.

The rest of my own work now falls into Era III medicine, the topic of the next chapter. In these cases I am working deep in the energy field, connecting with past lives and the ancestors, as well as those still living that we can connect with and impact through the universal energy field simply through intention and attention.

---

[87] The science of life, deriving from the Sanskrit terms ayur meaning life and veda meaning science or knowledge.
[88] Chopra, Deepak. 2005. Psychology of the Future: Lessons from Modern Consciousness Research, pp206-07 in *Consciousness and Healing* edited by Schlitz, Marilyn and Amorok, Tina with Micozzi, Marc S. St Louis, Missouri, USA: Elsevier

Chapter 10:
Non-local Medicine,
Era III Healing

'Integral medicine does not just refer to the science of diagnosing, treating or preventing disease and damage of the body or mind, but to a medicine that heals. It is a dynamic, holistic, life-long process that exists in widening and deepening relationships with self, culture and nature. Integral medicine is about transformation, growth and the restoration of wholeness. Health is seen not as the absence of disease, but as a process by which individuals maintain their ability to develop meaning systems that allow them to function, heal and grow in the face of changes in themselves, their relationships, and the world...
'The key to an integral approach is not the contents of the medical bag, but the holder of the bag – one who has opened herself to the multidimensional nature of healing, including body, mind, soul, spirit, culture and nature.' [89]
(Marilyn Schlitz)

In what Dossey defines as Era III medicine (see Chapter 9), mind is seen as unconfined by either space or time. It is recognised

---

[89] Schlitz, Marilyn. 2005. Preface: The Integral Impulse: An Emerging Model for Health and Healing, pp xl-xli in *Consciousness and Healing*, edited by Schlitz, Marilyn and Amorok, Tina with Micozzi, Marc S. St Louis, Missouri, USA: Elsevier

that our non-local mind may affect healing both within and between people. Non-contact healing modalities between people in each others' presence, as well as between people distant from each other, become possible with non-local mind, as do healings backwards and forwards in time.

The new medicines of psychoneuroimmunology, epigenetics and Era III healing have led to the construction of many new experiments testing the efficacy of how our own beliefs can impact our health and healing as well as testing the efficacy of how our thoughts and actions can impact the health and wellbeing of others, removed from us through either space, time or both.

Now that we are asking different questions and constructing these new experiments and studies, a mountain of evidence documenting our ability to control our own health is accumulating. A bit like quantum physics, it is being proven through experimentation, if not fully explained how, that all the various healings that tap into the energy fields, sheaths, nadis and chakras, such as Reiki, craniosacral therapy, vortex healing, theta healing, crystal therapy, emotional freedom technique, acupuncture, reflexology, prayer and spiritual healing are effective and are powerful complements to allopathic medicine and psychotherapy.

One interesting observation about the healings that emerged from the work of Robert Beck[90] as far back as the 1960s, is that all these Era III medicines appear to involve the healers' brains operating in a particular electromagnetic frequency range which is in alignment with the frequency of the Earth's magnetic field. Church reports Beck's work as follows. *'He performed experiments with healers from various regions and religions, including Amazonian shamans, Hawaiian kahunas, Christian faith healers, Indian yogis and Buddhist lamas, and showed that – at the moment of healing – their brain wave frequencies were virtually identical.*

'The Earth resonates at an average frequency of 7.8Hz, while the dominant brainwave frequency of sensitives, such as shamans and healers, comes close to 7.83 Hz, and may, at times, beat in

[90] Beck, Roberts. 1986. Mood modification with ELF magnetic fields: A preliminary exploration, p.4 *Archaues*

phase with the Earth's signal, thereby causing harmonic resonance...They appear to be tapping into a universal frequency that is implicated in healing, and is effective regardless of the belief structure of the healer.[91]

In *Healing Beyond the Body*, Dossey reports the results of many meta analyses of Era III medicines.[92] For instance, studies conducted over two decades at the Princeton Engineering Anomalies Research (PEAR) Laboratory show that non-local awareness operates through time as well as through space, showing odds against chance of one hundred billion to one that mentally sent images chosen at random from a computer data bank, are actually perceived by the 'receiver' precognitively up to several days before being sent and before being selected by the computer.

He reports, *'These results have been published in prestigious scientific journals such as Nature, proceedings of the IEEE, and the Journal of Scientific Exploration. Following his evaluation of the government-sponsored SAIC tests, Ray Hyman, the University of Oregon psychologist who is the most prominent critic of this field, conceded, 'I cannot provide suitable candidates for what flaws, if any, might be present.'*[93]

William Braud is another of the leaders in Era III testing. In *Transpersonal Images: Implications for Health*[94] he examines the evidence for the reality, validity and efficacy of non-local healings. In particular Braud is highly involved with testing the efficacy of experiments which appear to influence things that have already happened, retrospectively. He writes, *'We have also conducted sessions in which the to-be-influenced living system was distant in time. The procedures and analysis methods for these temporally nonlocal experiments are similar to those of*

---

[91] Church Ph.D., Dawson. 2007. *The Genie in Your Genes, Epigenetic Medicine and the New Biology of Intention.* pp 102-103 Llandeilo, U.K.: Cygnus Books

[92] Dossey, Dr., Larry. 2009. *Healing Beyond the Body.* pp 221-25 London, UK: Piatkus Books

[93] Dossey, Dr., Larry. 2009. *Healing Beyond the Body.* p.222 London, UK: Piatkus Books

[94] Braud, William. 2005. Transpersonal Images: Implications for Health. p.272 *Consciousness and Healing,* edited by Schlitz, Marilyn and Amorok, Tina with Micozzi, Marc S. St Louis, Missouri, USA: Elsevier

the concurrent influence studies, with the important difference that the activity of the living 'target' system was monitored and recorded before the influence attempts were made. Thus, any systematic results in such experiments involved time-displaced influences. Although such outcomes might seem to be impossible given conventional apprehensions of time and causality, there is nonetheless both theoretical and empirical support for such outcomes... Our imaginal processes appear to be capable of exerting objectively measurable influences not only upon present, distant biological and physical systems, but also upon the past and future activities of these systems.'[95]

The Soul Medicine Institute has set up the first international database of energy psychology case histories. This research tool collects medical and psychiatric diagnoses before treatment. It notes the energy psychology treatments used and the diagnosis after treatment. It is peer reviewed and conforms to the Consort Standards and the Standards of the National Institutes of Health.

In a book based on the results reported to the Institute[96], Dawson Church and Norman Shealy, M.D., Ph.D. document over one hundred scientific studies, and dozens of medically verified 'miraculous' cures, that demonstrate the power of thought, prayer and belief. They identify the three pillars of 'Soul Medicine' as being energy, intention and consciousness.

In *Prayer is Good Medicine*, Dr. Dossey reports that *'there are over 1200 scientific studies demonstrating the link between prayer and intention and health and longevity'.*[97]

Meta-analyses in the *Annals of Internal Medicine*[98] and *The*

[95] Braud, William. 2005. Transpersonal Images: Implications for Health, pp271-272 in *Consciousness and Healing*, edited by Schlitz, Marilyn and Amorok, Tina with Micozzi, Marc S. St Louis, Missouri, USA: Elsevier

[96] Shealy, M.D., Ph.D., Norman and Church Ph.D., Dawson 2008. *Soul Medicine: Awakening your Inner Blueprint for Abundant Health and Energy.* USA: Energy Psychology Press

[97] Dossey, Larry. 1997. *Prayer is Good Medicine.* p.104 New York, N.Y., USA: Harper Collins

[98] Astin, J.E., et al. 2000. The efficacy of 'distant healing': a systematic review of randomized trials. *Annals of Internal Medicine*, 132: p.903

Journal of Alternative and Complementary Medicine[99] have compiled the results of many studies and found that prayer, distant healing and intentionality have significant effects on healing.

In total these studies are illuminating the links between gene expression, electromagnetic energy transfer, quantum mechanics, string theory and human consciousness.

Lipton tries to explain how quantum entanglement not only allows for the possibility of energy healing, but negates a lot of what conventional medicine (Era I in the Dossey terminology) tries to achieve. In a conventional, causal, linear model, when something goes wrong you identify the malfunctioning step and by providing the malfunctioning cell with a functional replacement part for the faulty element, by prescribing a pharmaceutical drug for instance, the defective single point can theoretically be repaired and health restored.

'However, the quantum perspective reveals that the universe is an integration of interdependent energy fields that are entangled in a meshwork of interactions... A biological dysfunction may arise from a miscommunication along any of the routes of information flow. To adjust the chemistry of this complicated interactive system requires a lot more understanding than just adjusting one of the information pathway's components with a drug.'[100]

Because of the complexity of the interaction between different cells – possibly at far distant parts of the body – the results of the conventional focus on drug therapy are shocking. As Lipton reports, *'Adverse drug effects... are a primary reason why a leading cause of death is iatrogenic illness, ie illness resulting from medical treatment... Last year a new study, based on the results of a ten-year survey of government statistics [in the USA]... concludes that iatrogenic illness is actually the leading*

---

[99] Jonas, W.B. 2001. The middle way: Realistic randomized controlled trials for the evaluation of spiritual healing. *The Journal of Alternative and Complementary Medicine*, 7 (1): pp5-7

[100] Lipton Ph.D., Bruce H. 2005. *The Biology of Belief.* pp72-73 Carlsbad, CA, USA: Hay House, Inc.

cause of death in the United States and that adverse reactions to prescription drugs are responsible for more than 300,000 deaths a year.

'These are dismaying statistics, especially for a healing profession that has arrogantly dismissed three thousand years of effective Eastern medicine as unscientific, even though it is based on a deeper understanding of the universe. For thousands of years, long before Western scientists discovered the laws of quantum physics, Asians have honoured energy as the principal factor contributing to health and wellbeing.'[101]

He goes on to point out the failure of Western medical schools to include the mounting evidence on the effectiveness of Era III medicines in their curriculum.

'Hundreds upon hundreds of other scientific studies over the last fifty years have consistently revealed that 'invisible forces' of the electromagnetic spectrum profoundly impact every facet of biological regulation... Specific frequencies and patterns of electromagnetic radiation regulate DNA, RNA, and protein syntheses; alter protein shape and function; and control gene regulation, cell division, cell differentiation, morphogenesis (the process by which cells assemble into organs and tissues), hormone secretion and nerve growth and function. Each one of these cellular activities is a fundamental behaviour that contributes to the unfolding of life. Though these research studies have been published in some of the most respected mainstream biomedical journals, as of 2010 their revolutionary findings have not been incorporated into the medical school curriculum.'[102]

Is it all the placebo effect?

One possible explanation of Era II and Era III healings in current time could be the placebo effect. In *The placebo effect:*

---

[101] Lipton Ph.D., Bruce H. 2005. *The Biology of Belief.* p.77 Carlsbad, CA, USA: Hay House, Inc.
[102] Lipton Ph.D., Bruce H. 2005. *The Biology of Belief.* p.81 Carlsbad, CA, USA: Hay House, Inc.

illness and interpersonal healing[103], Miller, Colloca and Kaptchuk write, '*There is no standard definition of "the placebo effect". As a clinical phenomenon, "the placebo effect" is a generic name for beneficial effects that derive from the context of the clinical encounter, including the ritual of treatment and the clinician-patient relationship, as distinct from therapeutic benefits produced by the specific or characteristic pharmacological or physiological effects of medical interventions*'.

Western medicine has grappled for many years with the apparent power of the placebo effect (and of course the opposite, 'nocebo' effect, where patients get worse because they believe they will). Interestingly, if you type 'placebo' into the search engine of the US National Library of Medicine, you get 157,295 relevant articles, demonstrating its relevance to modern medicine and research!

Harris Dienstfrey, the founder and former editor of *Advances*, the journal of the Institute for the Advancement of Health, sums up the power of the placebo as follows. '*The long and short of the placebo phenomenon in drug studies is that the mind has an apparently limitless capacity to duplicate the results of whatever chemists concoct to relieve or resolve human ills and discomforts.*'[104]

I personally feel that the negative connotations generally associated with the word placebo are misplaced and actually I don't really care if people describe what I do as a placebo. On behalf of my clients all I care about is that their health and welfare improve.

What recent research is providing is the physiological explanation of **why** we do actually get better when we think we're getting better. Why when we believe something helps us it does. Why when we relax and become more positive our

---

[103] Miller, Franklin G., Colloca, Luana and Kaptchuk, Ted J. 2009 The Placebo Effect: Illness and Interpersonal Healing. *Perspectives in Biology and Medicine* Volume 52, Number 4, Autumn 2009. pp 518-39

[104] Dienstfrey, Harris. 2005. Mind and Mindlessness in Mind-Body Research, p.59 in *Consciousness and Healing*, edited by Schlitz, Marilyn and Amorok, Tina with Micozzi, Marc S. St Louis, Missouri, USA: Elsevier

endocrine and immune systems act in ways that improve our health. Era II physiology is demonstrating that we are largely in control of how our bodies function and their level of health (recognising that we are also largely, but not fully, in control of the environment we surround ourselves with, the food that we eat, the exercise that we engage in, the toxins that we use on our bodies and so on). This is our internal power, our potential, and if you want to think of it that way, yes, the power of the placebo.

Era III healings however still seem to be largely inexplicable in physiological terms and in terms of the placebo effect. In particular it is extremely difficult to see how the placebo effect could work backwards in time, to effect change in a group of people who didn't know they were the subject of a clinical trial. Similarly it is difficult to understand how the placebo effect could work for people in a coma or otherwise unaware they might be receiving any form of healing.

Once again it seems likely that the full explanation will emerge in the future from a greater understanding of the physics of non-locality. Targ is one person who has attempted to justify Era III medicine in terms of the continuity and non-locality of consciousness, the holographic universe. He says, '*We now know that our timeless awareness has mobility independent of our physical body. The evidence is very strong that awareness, which is what we are, can receive an inflow of information from all of space-time, and can generate an outflow of healing intention to the present, the future and the past. This all happens because space-time is nonlocal and there is no separation in consciousness.*'[105]

This is why, to me, it seems obvious that if we are to truly advance in our understanding of Era III medicine and our power to influence the health of ourselves and others by what we think (positively and negatively) as well as what we do, then healing professionals and quantum physicists have to communicate and work together. I believe we should all be searching for a new

---

[105] Targ, Russell. 2004. *Limitless Mind, a guide to remote viewing and transformation of consciousness.* p.101 Novato, CA, USA: New World Library

'unifying theory' which provides an explanation of the sub-atomic demonstrations of non-locality within linear accelerators and the macro-cosmic demonstrations of non-locality reported by distance healing through space and time.

Chapter 11:
Shamanism and the Ancient Traditions of Energy Healing in the South American Indians

'There may only be a few major healing themes in our entire lives, all of which stem from our original wounds. The rest of our psychic and physical aches and pains – no matter how devastating – are incidents that express these themes in different narrative forms. They're B movies made from the same script. When we come to understand this overarching theme, we can own it, break free of its plot, and become the authors of our own narrative'[106] (Dr. Alberto Villoldo)

The next step on my own journey into the worlds of energy and healing came with my shamanic training, which I embarked on in November 2007.

People often ask me what exactly is shamanism? The best answer I can give is that it is an ancient healing profession, practised by most of the indigenous peoples throughout the world. The most noticeable difference between shamans and

---

[106] Villoldo, Ph.D., Alberto. 2005. *Mending the Past and Healing the Future with Soul Retrieval.* pp51-52 Carlsbad, CA, USA: Hay House, Inc.

doctors is that whilst shamans, like doctors, have always been capable of dealing with physical ailments, they are also capable of seeing energetic ailments (including curses and psychic daggers) and are able to alter their state of consciousness to work outside linear space and time, enabling conversations with the spirits of the dead as well as animal, plant and earth spirits. In other words, they have always been able to access the non-local consciousness!

My initiation into shamanism came when I attended Dr. Alberto Villoldo's Light Body School. Dr. Villoldo himself was a classically trained medical anthropologist, until he was chosen by the Peruvian shamans to bring their healing techniques to the Western world.

This particular lineage of shamanism was kept very pure over many centuries, because when the conquistadors invaded Peru in the 1530s a group of the shamans fled to the high Andes to keep themselves and their traditions safe. There were myths and legends about the medicine men in the mountains, but for centuries they were never seen and they lived in total isolation. In 1949 a group of them came down from their hiding place in the mountains to join in the Festival of Qoyllur R'Iti, which is held annually near Cusco to coincide with the full moon at the end of May or the beginning of June. Stories tell of how the colourful, distinctive patterns of their woven clothes and their ponchos with the royal emblem of the sun made them immediately recognisable as the lost Incas, the 'Children of the Sun'. The stories add that an aisle parted in the crowd for them to pass through and the elders welcomed them, saying, *'We have been waiting for you for five hundred years.'*[107]

Villoldo lived and studied with the Peruvian shamans for twenty-five years, under the guidance of Don Antonio Morales. Today he runs the Four Winds Society[108] which offers trips to Peru and personal healings as well as the courses within the Light Body School. The initial Medicine Wheel programme spends a week working with each of the directions, starting in the South,

---

[107] I know it only appears to be four hundred years, but I am just reporting the legend!

[108] http://www.thefourwinds.com/

which focuses on shadow work, the pain and traumas that have been suppressed and your attachment to the past. Shadow work continues in the direction of the West, where you die to the old way of being and shed fear. In the North you drop your limiting roles and beliefs and learn to step outside space and time. In the East you learn how to work with energy and intention to create your own reality.

So how did Peruvian shamanism become my next form of encounter with altered states of consciousness, a different type of interaction with the universal energy?

Within a short space of time after starting to practise Reiki professionally, it became clear to me that I needed some sort of counselling qualification, as clients would go on the massage couch for body work after a brief initial conversation, but then would frequently become highly emotional as I was working with them, and as various types of traumas surfaced through the body contact and the flow of Reiki into the system. After finishing the body work, they would often want to talk about what had emerged, and I was working on a completely blank canvas in terms of counselling experience.

So it was that in 2007 I signed up for the Foundation year course at the Psychosynthesis & Education Trust[109], which teaches a highly transpersonal form of psychotherapy. The gifts I received from that year of training were huge, and I made some of my best friends through that course, but it became clear to me that the mind can dissemble for a long time and suppress painful memories into the shadows of the subconscious, whereas the body and the energy field do not hide their pain once given permission to express themselves. As a result, I decided that whilst counselling skills would be a necessary part of my energy and body work profession, I did not want to be a psychotherapist, based on talk and forbidden to make physical contact with my clients.

Indeed, whilst I understand that 'no touching' was a rule instigated to protect clients from unscrupulous therapists, it is a bit like the overly politically correct rules in place in nursery schools

---

[109] http://www.psychosynthesis.edu/

these days which prohibit teachers from hugging hurt children. In my belief we are in danger of creating another generation of emotionally damaged people who will suffer from abandonment issues and blurred physical boundaries because those put in positions of supposed care and responsibility cannot give children (and patients) that which they most need and desire at a young (or indeed any) age – physical connection and love, particularly in times of pain and stress. What many of my clients appreciate most about my bodywork therapy is just being held with an unconditional loving touch, in a safe space, being seen and heard and allowed to express whatever emerges – without judgement, without criticism. For psychotherapists to refrain from this physicality, to me, verges on further emotional abuse of the client.

Anyway, I digress...

Whilst researching books on 'core wounds' for the psychosynthesis course, in one of those fateful moments of my life, I stumbled across one of Villoldo's books, *Mending the Past and Healing the Future Through Soul Retrieval.* I had to buy it!

In it Villoldo says, '*although I'm trained both in psychology and the traditions of the Laika (the Peruvian shamans), I've found that one (shamanic) soul-retrieval session can accomplish what may take many years to heal employing psychotherapy. This is because to recover our innocence and trust in life we must renegotiate obsolete soul contracts and discard limiting beliefs, which happens during the soul retrieval journey. In addition the language of the soul is very different from what we use in therapy and counselling. It's rich in image, myth, archetypes and mystery – full of poetry and magic, it speaks to intuition and love. Abandonment, fear, insecurity and childhood trauma – all of these terms belong to the intellect. I'm convinced that when we only have these words to explain our childhoods, it's a sure sign that we're suffering from soul loss because the soul's very words have vanished.*'[110]

He explains more about the negative, limiting impact that old soul contracts can have on our lives. In my personal experience and from my work with clients, I know we can carry these old

---

[110] Villoldo, Ph.D., Alberto. 2005. *Mending the Past and Healing the Future with Soul Retrieval.* p.31 Carlsbad, CA, USA: Hay House, Inc.

soul contracts through many lifetimes, until we recognise the core wound that led us to write them in order to protect ourselves. At that point we can evaluate whether they still serve us. If not then we can re-write them and start to live life with a contract that is more useful to us at this time. As Villoldo puts it, *'More often than not, these pledges (the soul contracts) are made silently and honoured without discussion, or even consciousness, for many, many years. Although they may have worked well at the time of our wounding to create a sense of security in a world we deemed unsafe, they go on to become the source of our limiting beliefs about abundance, intimacy, love and success. In other words, a single soul contract will spawn dozens of limiting beliefs.'*[111]

As soon as read this, I was hooked! This was exactly the experience I had gone through at The Monroe Institute, when I needed to discard the contract I had written after being drowned as a witch, that *'From now on I will live in conformity with authority to protect myself and my family.'* I had to replace this with *'It is safe for me to step into my power and use my gifts'*.

Once more synchronicities were bringing together a variety of different underlying paradigms and teachings into a coherent whole, a unified healing path. Shamanism had to be my next exploration.

My first initiation came in November 2007 when I attended the first part of the Medicine Wheel, the South. The week long course took place in a beautiful country house hotel in Holland, surrounded by forests and rivers, where we could work with Mother Earth (Pacha Mama as she is known in South America).

The initial thing which surprised me, and also put my mind at rest, was the obvious intelligence and openness of the other participants. There was a high proportion of doctors and highly qualified medical professionals in the training group, as well as bankers, lawyers, IT specialists, management consultants and other professional people. Once again, as at the Monroe Institute, these were not 'new age hippies' but people seeking personal growth and development and a new way of being,

---

[111] Villoldo, Ph.D., Alberto. 2005. *Mending the Past and Healing the Future with Soul Retrieval.* p.64 Carlsbad, CA, USA: Hay House, Inc.

living in harmony with nature and in recognition that they were more than their physical bodies.

There were many profound healings for me that week, which was also amongst the toughest weeks of my life emotionally, but a particular highlight which I will always remember, was the first night of 'ritual'. At this ceremony, the four teachers were going to transmit to the students the first three rites of the Munay-Ki.[112] The basic principle underlying the Munay-Ki rites is that they transform and upgrade your energy field (the sheaths of the Indian tradition). They are energetic transmissions that help to heal the wounds of the past, i.e. your karmic and genetic inheritance.

The first rite, the Healer's Rite, awakens the healing power in your hands so that everyone you touch is blessed. The second rite, the Bands of Power, weaves five luminous belts into the luminous energy field for protection, breaking down any negative energy that comes toward you. The third rite, the Harmony Rite, transmits the qualities of the seven Archetypes into the Chakras. These are serpent, jaguar, hummingbird and eagle, plus the Keeper of the Lower World (our unconscious), the Keeper of the Middle World (our waking world), and the Protector of the Upper World (our superconscious). You can then perceive the world from any one of these very different perspectives. Serpent is a very grounded and literal place, jaguar allows emotional tracking and helps us to be fearless, hummingbird is joyful and represents the level of the individual soul whilst eagle sees the higher perspective, the big picture, from the level of the superconscious. We want to be able to access all levels of our consciousness clearly and with awareness: the frequently repressed unconscious, the reality of our everyday lives, and our potential, our connection with the non-local energy field or super-conscious. The Harmony Rite assists us in being able to switch perspectives in viewing any situation.

At seven o'clock on the night of the transmission of the first three rites we entered the room for the ceremony. It was candlelit and beautifully decorated with vegetation of all sorts. Ivy, pine branches, cones, shells, and stones, all representations

---

[112] For further information on the Munay-Ki rites see www.munay-ki.org

121

from Mother Earth, were spread around the room. Four places were set down the centre of the room where the teachers were sitting, dressed completely in black and surrounded by their ceremonial tools, known as mesas (the colourful cloths of the Peruvian shamans containing healing stones), feathers, bells, transmission stones and incense.

We all sat in a circle around the teachers and one by one we were given the rites through direct energetic transmission. I know it might sound like hocus pocus. But again my personal experience was hugely empowering. The teachers (one from the United States, one from Sweden and two from Holland) were chanting in Quechua, the language of the Quero people of the Andes, waving feathers and incense and ceremonial stones and shells. It felt so much like I was coming home – '*I am a witch, I have always been a witch, and in this lifetime that's OK!*' There was such relief. I was surrounded by supportive, intelligent, like-minded people, and we were all participating in powerful magic, powerful medicine, that in many past lives we would have been persecuted and possibly killed for. Now at last it felt truly safe to own and acknowledge and expand my power and my gifts, which have been repressed for so many lifetimes.

Initially, I went to the shamanic courses as a way of learning more about myself, healing myself, revisiting old and outdated contracts and rewriting them to come into my power, to accept my position as a co-creator of my own reality. I also expected to get 'tools' and processes that I could use with my clients, but increasingly it became evident to me that to be a shaman is not just about having a cool healing kit – it's a complete way of life.

The belief system that Villoldo teaches is entirely about empowerment, taking people out of the box of social conditioning, allowing them to step into their power, knowing they can impact their own destiny.

The core way of living is expressed by the opening I used for my morning meditation for a number of years, up until the time I started writing this book.

'May I live without attachment
May I live without fear
May I live without suffering
May I live without judgement
May I live in the way of beauty – seeing the beauty in all
people, all things, all situations
May I live with joy, saying 'yes' to life
May I live as love
May I live with gratitude – to mother earth and all she
provides, to all my teachers, for my health and for all
the many blessings in my life
Thank you, thank you, thank you for allowing me to sing
the song of life this day, in this body, on this beautiful
planet'

During the process of writing this book however, I came to the realisation that I only need the last three sentences of this prayer, as all the others are included automatically if I live with love. Love does not judge, love sees the beauty in everything, love has no suffering, no attachment, no fear.

One of the core beliefs of the shamanic path is that our problems stem from blockages in the luminous energy field, our everlasting energy, which reincarnates in different forms but never dies. Again this is in direct parallel to the chakra system and the energy sheaths described previously. The shamans are able to journey into this all-pervading luminous energy field, which is part of the infinite cosmos, for themselves and for others. In doing so, they travel outside conventional space and time. This is entirely consistent with the Indian philosophies of reincarnation and using meditation to open the kundalini channels to reach altered states of consciousness, spiritual evolution, clearing old karma and moving towards enlightenment.

As with yogic meditations, within shamanism and The Light Body School, many of the powerful healings I was taught depend on working with various altered states of consciousness, or journeying as it is labelled in the shamanic traditions.

The initial process is to go down into the subconscious, the place of repression and shadows, of pain, guilt, shame, anger. The intention is to cleanse yourself of these stored emotions and egotistical attachments. At a later stage, when the shadow work is complete, you can start to visit the superconscious, known in the shamanic tradition as the Upper World, the place where you attain your divine nature and learn about the true purpose of your life.

Villoldo says, 'Remember: *You journey to discover what's possible for your soul in this life and in the next. You journey to make sweeping changes, which can't be made in the small increments of daily life... The soul's choices are the great decisions that can only be made from the fifth plane, as you navigate through your destiny and express it in the now. In the Upper World, you'll be selecting your future – and all future incarnations to come.*'[113]

Once again the importance of every single moment, every single act is emphasised, for they impact our eternal future, lifetime after lifetime.

After the South and the West, the training steps into the direction of the North, the place on the Medicine Wheel at which trainees are really asked to step into living the way of the shaman.

At that point we are asked to bring four practices into our lives:

1. Beginner's mind – seeing things for the first time, making ourselves fresh for new experiences every day. Leading a simple life. Letting go of limiting beliefs, not identifying with our thoughts, letting every belief we hold about the nature of reality go to the fire. Engaging with life from a place of love, giving thanks for every moment.
2. Living consequently – knowing that every word, every thought, every action is energy moving and has a consequence – being aware of the ripples we create in time and taking responsibility for them.
3. The practice of transparency – allowing ourselves to be completely seen so there is nothing left to hide. Who we say we are is who we really are. Working on being valuable rather than popular. Living in awareness and stepping beyond the ego.

[113] Villoldo, Ph.D., Alberto. 2005. *Mending the Past and Healing the Future with Soul Retrieval.* p.159 Carlsbad, CA, USA: Hay House, Inc.

4. The practice of integrity – being true to our word and recognising its power to create reality. The more power we accumulate the deeper a hurtful word will go. And as we become more truthful, the more what we speak will come true.

Within the various training I did with Villoldo, I experienced a number of profound exercises, some of which are the basis of much of the work I now do with my clients.

One particularly tough experience for me was the 'death scene', which emerges in the final direction of the Medicine Wheel, the East. Working with my partner, who was taking on the role of shaman, whilst I was client, first I had to imagine sitting beside my 'river of life', noting what was unfinished business, still causing pain, unresolved. One of my huge regrets was that because of the way my children's father and I had both been brought up, with strong work ethics and little emotion, we had never given our children a carefree childhood. We didn't play out in nature with them, admiring the flowers, the trees and the rocks, we never went to a beach to splash in rock pools or fish, we never went camping or had bonfires or watched the stars. We had travelled with them to lots of exotic places to show them world cultures, but we had stayed in five star hotels and villas, with fancy restaurants, where they were probably bored rigid, had to 'behave themselves' and never got any sense of the local communities. Even the games we played with them were always designed to be educational, not fun.

Another of my regrets was not communicating better with my mother who died when I was eighteen. There is so much I don't know about her life and so much I could have learned – but the opportunity now has long passed.

Part of the purpose of the exercise is to ensure we no longer leave things undone – take the opportunities for healing and communication while they are available!

After the witnessing, the shaman does a full seven chakra illumination to release all the heavy energy that remains in this life. The last part of the exercise is pure psycho-drama, setting up the deathbed and working in groups of six. I chose to speak to both my children, my father, my aunt and my ex-lover, Sean, to say to each of them what needed to be said to heal any hurt or wounds between us before I died, to voice anything I had never been able to voice in life, to tell them anything I had never dared to say or tell.

It is another one of those exercises that must be experienced to be fully understood and appreciated. Each person who is standing in as representative for another, a person they have never met, gets incredibly accurate physical and emotional sensations, with words pouring through to the 'client' on the 'deathbed'. Highly charged and emotional conversations take place with the representatives standing in as the voices of the client's parents, grandparents, lovers, friend and children – allowing the healing of the unfaced and unspoken wounds that remain between the different people involved.

After everyone has been spoken to, the shaman then releases the client's energy aura to the light to be cleansed (using a special unwinding procedure) and after a couple of minutes, because it is an exercise during life rather than real death, brings the cleansed aura back and reconnects it to the physical body.

Working in our group of six people we enacted six death scenes in one evening. It was a hugely emotional experience for all those involved.

With a client, the psycho-drama deathbed section is missed out, but after the life review and the seven chakra illumination the aura is still taken off and cleansed, then reattached and manifestations are brought in regarding how to live from this moment forward: what is the soul's calling, its purpose? This proves to be a profound and life-changing exercise for most of the people I have been honoured to have shared this work with.

Another profound exercise during one of the advanced courses required partners to journey to see our biggest fear. Mine was about 'not knowing'. I had always felt I had to know 'how' everything works – in fact that has been one of the main driving forces for the journey described in this book. I had always felt that not knowing made me stupid or weak or vulnerable or not good enough.

As I have gone on this journey of exploration I have realised that in fact I hardly know anything and I control even less! That realisation has perversely been a huge relief for me. All we ever can **know** is that things are constantly changing and all we can **control** is how we react to events, not what others do and say or what happens in the world around us. So I can stop all my incessant doing and fixing and organising. Just be love. And watch my words. Be a lot more silent in my life.

Some of the messages I took home from that particular shamanic training week were that I can be soft, big, and funny. I can live as love. I can stop running around trying to fix things. I can surrender and trust. I don't need to **do** anything, I just need to **be** present and awake.

That frees up so much space in my life.

Chapter 12:
Peru and the Amazonian
Plant Medicine

'Ancient and aboriginal cultures have spent much time and energy developing powerful mind-altering techniques that can induce holotropic states. They combine in different ways: chanting, breathing, drumming, rhythmic dancing, fasting, social and sensory isolation, extreme physical pain, and other elements... Many cultures have used psychedelic plants for these purposes... Additional important triggers of holotropic experiences are various forms of systematic spiritual practice involving meditation, concentration, breathing and movement exercises, which are used in different systems of yoga, Vipassana or Zen Buddhism, Tibetan Vajrayana, Taoism, Christian mysticism, Sufism, or Cabalah.'[114] (Stanislav Grof)

Having trained with Villoldo in Europe, I deeply desired to go to Peru to meet the indigenous shamans and experience their country and their ways first hand.

---

[114] Grof, Stanislav. 2005. Psychology of the Future: Lessons from Modern Consciousness Research, p.250 in *Consciousness and Healing*, edited by Schlitz, Marilyn and Amorok, Tina with Micozzi, Marc S. St Louis, Missouri, USA: Elsevier

On my first trip in 2008, I worked with Jose Luis Herrara, who runs the Rainbow Jaguar Institute. I went with my daughter who was just sixteen at the time and we hiked the Andes in the company of Don Jose Luis and five other shamans from different tribes, as well as fourteen European and North American shamanic students. We visited a number of the ancient sacred Inca sites, doing ceremony at each of them and learning about the local cosmology.

The scenery of the Andes is breathtaking and amazing, but there were a couple of really difficult days for me physically, as much of the ten day hike was at an elevation of three to four thousand metres. I remember one particularly arduous trek from the river valley where we had camped for one night to the campsite at the sacred city of Choquequirao (three thousand and fifty metres), one of the last bastions of the Incas. Choquequirao is a two day trek from any town with a road and excavations did not start there until the 1970s. When we finally arrive we were camped on a steep slope below the ceremonial plateau and I was suffering from altitude sickness plus the cold. I kept slipping downhill in my tent as I tossed and turned, trying to get to sleep, but being unable to breathe very well and thinking I was about to die. Perversely, what finally allowed me to nod off was the thought that I was surrounded by amazing shamans, so that if I did die from my physical body that night they would take good care of my spirit! Suddenly my fear of dying left, allowing me to relax and actually keep myself safe and healthy.

The ceremonies we did on that trip were profound and beautiful, cementing the work I had already done with Villoldo and allowing my daughter also to become a mesa carrier (the mesa is the Andean healing bundle of the shamans).

On my second visit to Peru in 2010 I worked with a very different tradition of shamanism: that of the men and women of the Amazonian tribes whose life revolves around plant medicine. By this stage I thought I had worked through most of my shadows and karmic baggage, as well as having started ancestral healing, but the experiences of the plant medicine were at a very different intensity.

I turned up with George (my partner at that time) at Ashi

Meraya[115], a Shipibo Ayahuasca retreat centre for the diffusion and dissemination of Amazonian traditional plant medicine, immediately after quitting my corporate consultancy job in July 2010. During dry season Ashi Meraya is about an hour and a half by bumpy tuk-tuk from Iquitos, whose claim to fame is being the largest town in the world with no road connecting it to the outside world – you either have to get a boat down the Amazon from Brazil, or fly in from Lima. I flew. In wet season you had better have wellies, as you will be wading along the muddy stream that the path degenerates into shortly after leaving the town, with your rucksack on your back. In dry season you have the luxury of the tuk-tuk ride.

For centuries many of the shamans around the world have used hallucinogenic plants to help in their journeying. Indeed the shamans of the Andes are unusual in **not** working with hallucinogens. These plant medicines have been prohibited in our Western society. We have illegitimised them whilst retaining the violence and addiction producing legalised drugs of alcohol and manufactured, chemically enhanced cigarettes.

George and I went to Ashi Meraya for a two week intensive immersion experience into the mysteries of plant medicine. Our bamboo hut was in a jungle clearing, on stilts, with a thatched roof. The toilet and shower were on the other side of the clearing, an area that the large Amazonian frogs and toads particularly liked to sit in during the dark hours. I have always had a fear of both rodents and toads, so the combination of creatures who nested in the thatched roof running across the bamboo rafters in the early hours of the morning, and the prospect of squishing a toad as I went to the toilet with extreme diarrhoea after the plant medicine ceremonies was not conducive to sleeping soundly. Nevertheless, I survived, and I would totally recommend Ashi Meraya to anyone who wants to experience the plant medicine in a safe, held, respectful, knowledgeable setting with amazing friendliness and hospitality.

The centre offers retreats lasting between two weeks and six

---

[115]http://www.elmundomagico.org/ashi-meraya-centre-of-traditional-amazonian-medicine/

months, so we were on one of the shortest possible visits. The longer retreats teach participants about hundreds of the Amazonian plants, explaining how to identify them, pick them and to use them, separately and in combination, to heal many kinds of disease. People who go on the longer retreats work with different types of plants in turn, but always including ayahuasca ceremonies, with the ayahuasca brew considered to be a powerful combination of some of the most powerful 'master plants'.

On our visit, our ayahuascero was Don Alfredo, a diminutive man from the Shipibo ethnic group. He has lived and worked in the jungle with the plants all his life. He explained to us that the body absorbs the energy of the plant medicine, which cleans us inside by drawing out the heavy energy. The spirit of the ayahuasca brew is multiple and it may appear as an animal or as a person. It is a very powerful medicine, chemically based on di-methyltriptamine (DMT) (which has more recently been named by scientists as the 'spirit molecule'), in combination with a monoamine oxidase inhibitor (MAOI). It clears and cleanses the body, both physically and spiritually.

Don Alfredo was very persistent that before each ceremony we needed to be clear on our intention for the evening. He asks all participants to concentrate and focus their intention in the moments they feel the ayahuasca taking hold. My questions included: what am I looking for? What do I need to release? How should I be living my life? The shamans believe the ayahuasca will teach you everything you ask for. They are there with you in each ceremony, helping to cleanse and heal.

It is also vital that you follow a very restricted diet during the time you are working with ayahuasca – no dairy products, no red meat, no alcohol, no coffee and no sexual activity. There is strong science behind this as MAOIs in conjunction with certain foods can produce very damaging side effects.

On the eight days when we were going to do ceremony in the evening, we had breakfast of fruit and eggs and herbal tea, then a very light lunch of vegetable soup and tea and nothing else except water until the ceremony at eight o'clock in the evening. One reason for this is that you want the stomach to be relatively empty in order to get the full absorption of the plant medicine. The other reason is that the ayahuasca is a huge cleansing agent and you nearly always vomit, hence the less that is in the stomach the better.

The ceremonies themselves take place at an isolated 'temple' in the middle of the jungle. Each time we followed a raised wooden walkway through the rain forest, walking for about fifteen minutes surrounded by the evening cacophony of noise from the thousands of species of birds, insects and monkeys that inhabit the area. The first time Don Alfredo carefully showed us the tarantula nests along the side of the path, so we would know where they were and what they looked like. They are not something you want to step on by accident as you return to your jungle hut in a hallucinogenic haze!

Inside the temple itself there were mats and cushions and vomit basins around the edge of the circle. We were extremely fortunate in that there were only two other guests at Ashi Meera while we were there, so there were just four of us, plus the shaman and his wife and an interpreter, during the ceremonies.

On each occasion, Don Alfredo would open the sacred space and then give each of us what he judged to be the right amount of the ayahuasca based brew. Each shaman uses a slightly different recipe, but Don Alfredo's particular brew included the DMT containing chacruna, the ayahuasca vine itself (containing the MAOI), and also toe, huambisa and bobinsana. The first couple of nights we were drinking a brew he had made previously, but from the third ceremony onwards, we were drinking a brew we ourselves had helped to make by pounding the hard, wooden stems of the freshly cut vines to soften them, before boiling them in water over a fire for several hours along with the other plants which activate and enhance the ayahuasca brew's impact.

The resulting concoction is thick and dark brown, with a very distinctive, woody taste and smell. I could only drink it in tiny sips, almost gagging each time, and it turned out that I only needed about half a cup to get the best effect, although others would drink two full cups – it depends on each person's individual system and the shaman's deep ability to see what is appropriate for each person.

Throughout all of the ceremonies Don Alfredo and his wife would sing the Icaros, the special songs that call in the plant medicine and help to release the heavy energy in a safe way, bringing in protection and cleansing and healing. These songs are unlike anything else I have ever heard and come through every shaman in a direct transmission from the plants themselves. Don Alfredo was a tiny man physically, but when he sang he sounded like a giant, with a huge, amazingly powerful tone that would fill the ceremonial space.

The following extracts are taken from the journal I kept at the time, and I hope they give a sense of the information and experience that I had of ayahuasca.

Ceremony 1 – Took the ayahuasca for the first time last night and it was really not a very pleasant experience! Gut-wrenchingly sick. I felt possessed and immobile, incapable of action. I just wanted it to stop. I asked the ayahuasca to show me something positive, to encourage me to do it again, but nothing came. I just got red and white lights and a swirling vortex, but I didn't go down into it. My body felt numbingly heavy and tired, I really struggled to stay awake.

Ceremony 2 – Full cup of ayahuasca and then just massive purging. Several different phases. In the first phase I felt I was totally losing control, I couldn't move my body or influence what was happening. There was lots of fear. I could see an orange 'operating room' tunnel in front of my head and some kind of a doctor kept coming in with trays of stuff to put into my head. It felt like total overload in my head.

Then there was the first vomiting phase. I wasn't seeing so many visions, just darkness spewing out of me, over and over and over. It was everything toxic in my system, my own stuff and the heavy energy which I had taken in from my clients over the years, all releasing from me. I lay down and Don Alfredo was cleansing me with Florida water[116] with his hands pulling from my belly, removing heavy energy from there. Then it felt as if my left hand had something stuck in it that needed to be taken out. George called Don Alfredo over again to remove whatever entity was there.

---

[116] Florida water is a combination of alcohol and herbs and is used throughout Peru for cleansing the energy field. The shamans usually take a swig of it and then blow it out in a fine spray over the area that needs purification.

In the third phase I was lying with my head in George's lap before sitting up next to him. I couldn't bear to have his hands on me to begin with as it felt as if there were so many other hands working on me from a different dimension, so I needed to keep human hands off me until that other work was finished. I was shaking uncontrollably a lot of the time and sweating, like having a massive fever. Then the whole of my female genealogical lineage came to me and their pain came out through me for healing. I was screaming and screaming and screaming uncontrollably, interspersed with vomiting, but although it was very powerful and emotional it was very distinctively not my own pain, it was all women's pain. That subsided after a while, but my mother was still left standing right in front of me, needing something, so once again Don Alfredo came over and gave her spirit whatever healing it needed.

The fourth phase was gradually coming out of the hallucinogenic state and back into my own body. It took a while. I had to go out of the temple and stand connecting with the earth, grounding myself then holding onto a tree to feel as if I was in my body and for a while, every time I closed my eyes, waves of shaking and sweating and the swirling lights came back, seeming to drag me out of my body again, but gradually I got grounded.

I definitely got cleansing for both myself and my clients. I need to consider how to keep myself clean in future and not take in other people's darkness. I thought I used extensive protection, but it doesn't seem to be enough.

Ceremony 4 – This time I just drank half a cup of ayahuasca. Some of the clear visions were of spirits working around the second chakra, particularly on the left-hand side. They seemed to be cutting cords. Also at one point I seemed to be lying in a leafy cocoon with a network or web around me, whilst beings were doing some sort of programming or healing. I had a very vivid image of a cat's face. I didn't vomit during the ceremony, although quite a lot of waves were going through my body and I was shaking again. It felt as if stuff was being released.

When I got back to the hut after the ceremony I was very sick. Then when we went to bed I was guided to work with one hand on George's head and one hand on his left shoulder. There was an amazing vision behind his head, like a sound board wall covered with nodules, with sort of white anemone type plants with waving tendrils emitting energy through my hands into George. Next day the frozen shoulder he has had for several years was ninety percent better! I also got a vision during the night of a big, pointy leaf plant coming out from the ground with a huge stem up the middle and a vibrating light on the top – again this was energy coming through me and into George. I was aware of travelling quite far 'out of body' because I had several shock landings back 'in', although I have no clear recollection of what happened out there, but lots of work seemed to be done on me. The Maestro says the three major jungle spirits came into the room during the ceremony to work on my abdomen and clear stuff the ayahuasca couldn't shift.

Ceremony 5 – Yesterday's ceremony was incredibly powerful for both of us. I would have felt completely overwhelmed if I didn't understand the process a little more now. Such vivid, intense, varied visions. Near the beginning some old women, 'the grandmothers', were walking across a bridge toward me. Then a young woman came and worked on me. Then I got taken outside the room into a tent where the whole 'family' were working on me as I lay on a table. Then another youngish man appeared and stood by my right-hand side for what seemed like a long time.

There was also quite an intense dark spell when Don Alfredo seemed to have shape-shifted into a huge yellow lizard type creature on the forest floor. He came over to stand right in front of us. He seemed to be calling something out of me and I was vomiting it up as he worked there. Don Alfredo's voice was huge. He is such a little man physically with such a big voice and such power.

Later I was in a huge vaulted cathedral-like space with a white, red and blue network of incredibly bright lights shining down from the ceiling. They formed a web of light above me. It was the most beautiful thing I had ever seen but almost overpowering. Towards the end of the ceremony Don Alfredo came over and blew down through my chakras from the crown, cleansed my face and aura extensively with Florida water, then had me hold the Florida water and breathe deeply three times through the right then the left nostril to complete my cleansing.

Ceremony 8 – Last day! Had a wonderful ceremony last night. It was slow to kick in for me and I had been holding on to my intentions of healing my relationships with family, healing my feet, asking for guidance on where and how I should be working. Nothing was happening, so eventually I just lay down and felt disappointed since it was the last night, but I accepted that nothing was going to emerge. As soon as I did that and surrendered, this brilliant white, glowing 'spider' landed right on my third eye and started building a pulsing network across my brain. I felt as if it was opening the pineal gland. It seemed to be totally opening my compassion. It was incredibly powerful and beautiful and in those moments it really felt as if that was why I was here – that would have been enough just on its own.

I felt at one point as if I was being pressed down on and almost immobilised by something very heavy. It was almost the feeling that I was being anaesthetised, and then some other orange 'insect' came out of a big orange tree trunk and again was working on my forehead and pineal gland. Then I got very shivery and shaky as usual.

Finally I went over to George to let him hold me and as we were sitting together I looked up and it was as if we were sitting underground, surrounded by the roots of a huge tree, and I was looking up the inside of the trunk and this amazing white light was coming down the inside of the trunk and surrounding both of us.

To close the ceremony we all had to stand up while Don Alfredo was singing the closing icaros. Don Alfredo said afterwards the spider was the ayahuasca and it was now inside me to help me with my clients. He said the heaviness I felt was when he was putting his protection into and around me. The big tree was remokaspi, another of the master plants, which is a very powerful force for me.

Lessons

One of the really interesting things for me is that although I was in many ways 'out of control' of both my body and my mind during these experiences, I still to this day have totally clear recall of the images I received during the ayahuasca ceremonies which is totally unlike the oblivion that can result from excessive alcohol. Clarity and memory are totally unimpaired by taking ayahuasca. It results in enhanced, not diminished, visualisation and awareness.

I felt totally cleansed at the end of the retreat, of my own pain, of the heavy energy that I had unknowingly taken in from my clients and of much ancestral pain. Not only had I benefitted myself, but I had helped clear the heavy energy that my genetic ancestors had carried for years.

Unfortunately, the authorities in the USA and the UK have deemed that ayahuasca is an illegal drug, and so the only plant medicine ceremonies that take place in the UK are illicit and not well advertised. As a result, there has been very little real investigation of the way that plant medicine impacts the brain and the information it helps to convey. The most notable investigation is described below.

The links between DNA, DMT, energy healing and the cosmic consciousness

Jeremy Narby is a Doctor of Anthropology from Stanford University. He lived in the Peruvian Amazon for two years, studying the Ashaninca Indians and became fascinated by their knowledge of the healing properties of plants. He kept being told the knowledge came from the plants themselves, particularly during ayahuasca ceremonies, such as those I have just described.

Each ayahuasca shaman has his or her own particular brew, but in all cases the primary hallucinogenic substance is the dimethyltryptamine (DMT) contained in the chacruna plant, made effective by being combined with the MAOI contained in the banisteriopsis caapi vine, commonly known as ayahuasca.

As Narby writes in *The Cosmic Serpent*, '*So here are people without electron microscopes who choose, among some 80,000 Amazonian plant species, the leaves of a bush containing a hallucinogenic brain hormone, which they combine with a vine containing substances that inactivate an enzyme of the digestive tract, which would otherwise block the hallucinogenic effect. And they do this to modify their consciousness.*

'It is as if they knew about the molecular properties of plants and the art of combining them, and when one asks them how they know these things, they say their knowledge comes directly from hallucinogenic plants.'[117]

Narby himself experimented with ayahuasca and became convinced that the plant medicine really did communicate information, so he then dedicated the next few years of his life to seeking the scientific explanation for how this could be possible. His research chronicles the multitude of indigenous peoples whose cosmological myths are based on the serpent or the dragon – sometimes an individual creature, but more often a twinned or double serpent, sometimes with wings, which can represent a variety of myths. He gradually connects the twin serpents of mythology, to the double helix of DNA.

He reaches the conclusion that DNA is at the origin of shamanic knowledge, and that by various methods the shamans around the world induce neurological changes that allow them to pick up information from the DNA present in the cells of all living beings. However, he knew of no neurological mechanism on which to base this hypothesis, but he did know that DNA was an aperiodic crystal that traps and transports electrons with efficiency and that emits photons (in other words, electromagnetic waves) at ultra-weak levels currently at the limits of measurement.

So, DNA is the source of the photon emission that comes from the cells of all living beings. The wavelength at which DNA emits these photons corresponds exactly to the narrow band of visible light, with its spectral distribution ranging at least from infrared (at about nine hundred nanometers) to ultraviolet (up to about two hundred nanometres). This photon emission has a high degree of coherence, meaning that it gives the sensation of bright colours, a luminescence and an impression of holographic depth.

---

[117] Narby, Jeremy. 1999. *The Cosmic Serpent, DNA and the Origins of Knowledge.* pp10-11 New York, NY, USA: Jeremy P. Tarcher/Putnam

He concludes that *'the molecules of nicotine or dimethyltryptamine, contained in tobacco or ayahuasca, activate their respective receptors, which set off a cascade of electrochemical reactions inside the neurones, leading to the stimulation of DNA and more particularly to its emission of visible waves, which shamans perceive as 'hallucinations'.'* [118]

He went on to look in the biophoton literature for a link between these DNA emitted photons and consciousness. He couldn't find any publication dealing with this connection, so he called Fritz-Albert Popp [119] in Germany and asked if he had considered the possibility of a connection between DNA's photon emission and consciousness. Popp told him, *'Yes, consciousness could be the electromagnetic field constituted by the sum of these emissions. But, as you know, our understanding of the neurological basis of consciousness is still very limited.'* [120]

However, Narby's hypothesis requires that DNA should be a photon **receptor** as well as an emitter. Within the DNA structure, the four bases stack up on top of each other in the order dictated by the genetic text, giving it an aperiodic structure. *'However, this is not the case for the repeat sequences that make up a full third of the genome... In these sequences, DNA becomes a regular arrangement of atoms, a periodic crystal – which could, by analogy with quartz, pick up as many photons as it emits. The variation in the length of the repeat sequences, (some of which contain up to 300 bases) would help pick up different frequencies and could thereby constitute a possible function and new function for a part of 'junk' DNA.'* [121] (That junk accounts for a massive ninety-seven percent of our DNA!)

Back in Chapter 3, when discussing the implications of the

---

[118] Narby, Jeremy. 1999. *The Cosmic Serpent, DNA and the Origins of Knowledge.* p.127 New York, NY, USA: Jeremy P. Tarcher/Putnam

[119] A German physicist and founder of the International Institute of Biophysics in Neuss, Germany, credited with the discovery of biophoton emissions – tiny currents of light emanating from living things.

[120] Narby, Jeremy. 1999. *The Cosmic Serpent, DNA and the Origins of Knowledge.* p.128 New York, NY, USA: Jeremy P. Tarcher/Putnam

[121] Narby, Jeremy. 1999. *The Cosmic Serpent, DNA and the Origins of Knowledge.* p.130 New York, NY, USA: Jeremy P. Tarcher/Putnam

holographic universe, I said that metaphorically we have to become like the right light source to illuminate the information contained in the hologram, which means sending out the right waves to access or connect with the holographic universe. This work by Narby seems to suggest that our DNA is the 'right light source', particularly when stimulated by a chemical such as DMT. If we could all learn to activate our pineal glands to produce DMT endogenously, as highly experienced meditators are able to do, then we could all have much greater access to the inforealm whenever we wanted!

I am not aware of any studies of the receptor properties of biophotons and DNA and this is clearly an area where future research is needed if we are truly to understand how to access the wisdom of plant medicine. I would ask any reader who has more recent research on this to please let me know at *balanceandpurposehealing@gmail.com*.

I would like to finish by saying that from my personal experience ayahuasca is most definitely **not** a recreational drug. It is an amazingly strong journeying tool, **only** to be used under the supervision of a qualified shaman who is able to hold the space, to conduct the rituals with respect, to talk to the plants, to see the energies of the plants and all the participants in the ceremony (physical and non-physical) and deal with the frequently deep pain that may emerge and subsequent healing that can result. But if you can avail yourself of that experience, it is something that is likely to change your life and your belief system forever.

Chapter 13:

Accessing the Universal Energy Field through Love and Tantric Yoga

'Love is the experience of oneness... Love is the experience
when the walls between two people have crumbled down and
their beings have met, united and become one. When this
experience happens between two individuals I call it love.
When this same experience happens between an individual and
the whole, I call that experience godliness.'[122] (Osho)

So far in my personal story, I have focused on the energetic
awareness that I was experiencing and learning to use through
the various altered states of consciousness and journeying that I
was experimenting with, but this was accompanied by a gradual
realisation of my transpersonal or 'Higher Self'. In many different
schools of philosophy and metaphysics this Higher Self is part
of the universal energy, however you want to label or define that
(for instance, God or consciousness), and the intention of
meditation is frequently to let go of duality between our ego and
the universal energy, to reach a state of Oneness with whatever
you perceive that external force to be.

---

[122] Osho. 1973. *From Sex to Superconsciousness.* pp37-38 Pune, MS, India:
Osho Media International

Love is seen as the first step to Oneness, also labelled Gnosis or awareness. And in order to love others, most great ancient philosophies and modern psychologies agree that first of all you need to learn to love yourself. The exception perhaps is Christianity, with many preachers continuing to teach that all human beings are sinners, particularly women, who are still blamed for the expulsion of Adam and Eve from the Garden of Eden. And Mary Magdalene is often still portrayed as a prostitute rather than as the leading disciple and likely the wife of Christ.

However, as most psychologists and psychotherapists know only too well from the string of clients that they see, most of us do **not** love ourselves. In fact many of us have been conditioned to be afraid of our magnificence. In the Western world we have often become our own harshest critics. Psychotherapists frequently work with the client's inner judge or inner critic sub-personality. I find that there are two core beliefs that are prevalent in the vast majority of my clients: either 'no-one loves me'; or, even more damaging, 'I am unlovable'. This may come from our childhood, when we experienced abandonment of many different types, intentional or otherwise, by our caretakers. It may come from karma and contracts we carry into this lifetime from previous lives. And it may come from the genealogical lineage, the collective unconscious of the culture and the family that we chose to be born into.

Self compassion starts by admitting our own frailty and being able to reach out and ask for help. But this often seems frightening and risky. What if we are rejected; what if we fail; what will other people think; how might others take advantage of our weakness? This is particularly true for those of us who have asked for help in the past and been disappointed or worse.

There are hundreds of books written on the philosophical objective of learning to love ourselves, ranging across self help manuals, psychotherapy texts, spiritual teachings and sex books.

In the Western world a lot of problems around self love appear to stem from underlying guilt and shame about our sexuality. Unfortunately much of this guilt and shame stems from a variety of religions which have frequently been dominated and controlled by men and hence have been particularly worried about the sexual power and energy of women. But of course sexual energy is one of the strongest drivers of the human condition and turning it from something beautiful and joyful into something shameful and disgusting doesn't make it disappear! Suppression, misunderstanding and misuse of sexual energy leads to pain, unhappiness, anger and blame within relationships, as well as the societal problems associated with pornography, rape, sexual abuse, sexual mutilation and sexual degradation.

Sensuality and sexuality are very different and physical touch is a vital part of human communication and nurturing, but touch has become so abused and confused with a self-serving, grasping form of sexuality that people are terrified to reach out physically to each other. This adds to the sense of alienation and aloneness that people feel in a society where communities and families have frequently disintegrated.

Another huge part of the healing I was receiving and the lessons I was learning as I worked with my various teachers was in connection with my own repressed sexuality which was very much associated with my conditioning about morality, ethics and the Christian version of God.

So, how did I get from where I was to a place of self love and acceptance of my divine sexuality?

It was thanks to many people I met along the healing path, teachers, friends and lovers, who helped me to reach into my personal shadows, acknowledge them and release them with gratitude for the lessons and gifts they had provided me with. It was also through discovering the ancient healing art of tantra, which helped me to reclaim my sacred feminine energy as a human manifestation of the Divine Mother, the Goddess, the creator of life, the One?

But I am getting ahead of myself – I was not ready for tantra in the initial stages – much other 'shadow' work was necessary first. Any shadow work of course is painful at the time, but the shadows are there whether acknowledged or repressed. From my own personal work and my work with clients, I truly believe that it is their repression that makes us sick in the long term.

Today, much of the work I do with clients is acknowledging that part of being human is acknowledging and accepting that 'shit happens'. However, we don't need to get weighed down by carrying an increasingly heavy bag of shit around with us. We need to look at the shit, acknowledge it, and either integrate the gifts and the lessons the experience has given us or let it go, releasing it from our energy field and releasing the limiting beliefs that are almost always attached to it.

One of my shadows had been a denial of emotions and the beauty and power of being a woman. I had been living from a very left-brain, masculine perspective. Anything one of the boys could do, I could do better. I had totally repressed my feminine, creative, nurturing, compassionate side, including my sexuality.

Since 2005 the various trainings I have undertaken have involved gradual sexual liberation, realising that making love to a beloved is as close to unity both with another human being and with the divine as we can experience in a human body. I learned that sacred sex is a hugely joyous experience, involving far more than genital stimulation. It is a complete energetic transfer and bonding with the beloved.

I have come to understand that once we honour all human beings as the Divine Masculine and the Divine Feminine having a human experience, then when we make love with our beloved, we are making love with and honouring the Divine which exists in every human form.

If we see the Divine in all humanity it also makes it impossible for us to intentionally inflict pain upon another – including sexual activities such as pornography, child abuse, rape and domestic violence, as well as wider abuses of one human being by another, including torture and murder.

I also gradually realised that true love and compassion are unconditional. The love I had received in my life until then appeared to have been conditional... I will love you if you do this. I won't love you if you do that. I will love you if you behave this way. I won't love you if you behave that way.

The first step on this path came immediately after my first rebirthing experience. When I finally came around, I had several long telephone conversations with Sean, who had collected me from Deike's and stayed with me until I was sufficiently grounded to drive home, collecting my daughter en route. I had been thinking of him a lot and had discussed with several friends how lucky I had been that someone so trustworthy had helped me. Given the state I had been in when he collected me, he could have robbed, raped or simply abandoned me and I would have had no recall of the event. I had thanked him profusely on the phone and he had just laughed and said not to be silly, it had not been a problem.

Trust was a big issue for me at that time as the result of a previous relationship with a chronic liar, who could never be relied upon, but I realised that because he had not taken advantage of my vulnerability, I did trust Sean.

A few days before my birthday, I e-mailed him to see if he wanted to go out in London that weekend, to make up for me being so incoherent on our previous meeting. He was coming to town anyway for another meeting during the day, so we arranged that he would come to my house on Saturday evening and we would go out to my favourite jazz club.

That night, with the affirmation I had just completed flashing through my mind, 'It is now safe for me to ask for what I want', combined with the incredible feeling of trust I had developed as a result of his taking care of me, I asked him to spend the night with me and he accepted. That was the start of a relationship which lasted almost two years. We were both absolutely convinced that destiny had guided us to sit next to each other at the Remote Viewing course the previous November and then to keep in touch for a particular purpose in this life, and that it is not the first life time in which we have been together.

Despite our attraction for each other and the deep love we both felt, Sean was nevertheless convinced right from the start of our relationship that we would not be together forever. He believed strongly that we had been brought together for a brief journey, recognising each other as part of an ongoing soul group needing help. But he also felt the love we shared would be temporary and that after we had helped each other our paths would diverge again. So there was a purpose in our being brought together at a time of need: we would help to heal each other, help each other to find a new path and then move on.

His prediction turned out to be entirely accurate. Some two years later he travelled to the United States to work with a group of Native Americans and shamans and there he met another woman that he fell in love with and is now married to.

At the time I was devastated! I went into the only real depression I have experienced in my life, but fortunately at the same time I was starting the Foundation Course in psychosynthesis. The support and teachings I received there helped me through that painful time, guiding me towards seeing the lessons and gifts of the relationship that had just ended, rather than getting stuck in the pain, rejection and abandonment.

I gradually realised that I had begun to use Sean as a crutch, as a support, as a man who would look after me and make my life easier by sharing in everyday chores like driving and fixing things around the house. I had also put him on a pedestal as my spiritual teacher and 'guru'. I had handed too much of my power to him and given him too much responsibility for my life. I saw that I had to make my own choices, set my own objectives and come up with my own path, independent of him, if I was to grow and develop in the way I was supposed to. He loved me and had always recognised this. His intention had always been for me to develop into my true self, to become all I am capable of being.

The experience also led me to realise that because I had lived such an emotionally suppressed life, truly feeling unconditional love for and from another and then the acute pain of loss, was exactly what I needed. For forty-five years I had been taught to live in equanimity, without expressing sorrow or joy, repressing my true self, my anger, my sexuality, my love, my neediness, my pain. I needed the high and then the crashing low to awaken and to truly say 'yes' to life, to living each moment, experiencing each moment and becoming conscious rather than asleep.

With hindsight now, some years later, I know absolutely that we were not destined to be together for a prolonged period. It would have been limiting if we had stayed together. We gave each other immense gifts and lessons. I love him still and think of him with enormous gratitude. But the next growth, the next part of the journey, had to bring in tantra, a discipline that Sean was not interested in. And I needed to learn to be OK by myself, not dependent on a man or societal approval for happiness.

It would not be until 2010 that I came across Osho, whose work I now quote frequently with my clients and who seems to express it perfectly.

In *New Man for the New Millennium* he talks on the theme that love for others is only possible when you have already achieved self love. '*The capacity to be alone is the capacity to love. It may look paradoxical to you, but it is not. It is an existential truth: only those people who are capable of being alone are capable of love, of sharing, of going into the deepest core of the other person – without possessing the other, without becoming dependent on the other, without reducing the other to a thing, and without becoming addicted to the other. They allow the other absolute freedom, because they know that if the other leaves, they will be as happy as they are now. Their happiness cannot be taken by the other, because it is not given by the other.*

'*Then why do they want to be together? It is no longer a need, it is a luxury. Try to understand it. Real persons love each other as a luxury; it is not a need. They enjoy sharing: they have so much joy, they would like to pour it into somebody. And they know how to play their life as a solo instrument.*' [123]

Unfortunately, the vast majority of relationships seem to be built on co-dependency at best or a perception of 'ownership' at worst. And many people are still stuck in desperately unhappy, unloving and damaging relationships by the religious vows of marriage and the legal/financial ties that accompany these, whether that is in their best interests or not. Such relationships frequently don't allow growth, self-expression, freedom or love.

Coming back to my personal story, there was a profound afternoon during the psychosynthesis course when we had to draw our major sexual block and then do Gestalt work[124] with it, talking to it and sitting in its place, allowing it to respond, to and fro, until a resolution was reached. My block was a traditional 'Old Testament', judgemental, critical God who will condemn me to hell if I sin. After a very difficult the resolution

---

[123] Osho. 2000. *New Man for the New Millennium.* pp 130-131 Osho International Foundation

[124] Gestalt therapy was founded by Frederick and Laura Perls in the 1940s. It is a philosophical study of the structures of subjective experience and consciousness, within which patients and therapists dialogue, that is, communicate their subjective perspectives of what is actually being done, thought and felt in the present moment.

in this case was to rip my drawing into shreds. That was no longer my God. That was the God of my childhood, but my 'God' is compassionate, forgiving and above all, loving.

When I truly accepted this into my energy field, and let go of the guilt and shame around sex that had accompanied me that far, I was ready for tantra. There is a Buddhist teaching that says when the student is ready the teacher will arrive. He did!

The next hugely significant lover and partner in my life was George, a beautiful, creative, artistic musician and photographer (mentioned previously as my fellow traveller and support on my trip to the Amazon to work with the plant medicine). He introduced me to the sacred yoga of tantra, a path I have been following ever since, with a variety of amazing professional teachers, including Ma Ananda Sarita that I worked with at Osho Nisarga in Northern India[125], John Hawken that I have worked with (along with George) in London[126] and Martin and Hanna of *Transcendence: authentic tantric yoga*, that I have worked with both in London and at their tantric temple in Wiltshire[127]. I have done singles workshops, couples workshops and private sessions on my own and with a partner.

Tantra is unique in accepting and embracing our sexuality within a philosophical tradition, but it is not purely sexual, as often portrayed in the Western media. It is a yoga practice based on the Divine Masculine and Feminine. We all contain masculine and feminine elements within ourselves, and many times we suppress one or the other (or even both). I had repressed the feminine for far too long, depending on my own masculine energy and yet also (paradoxically) needing constant approval from an external man in order to feel good about myself.

To heal and come into our magnificence, we need to recognise and harmonise our masculine and feminine essences and tantric yoga is a profound and ancient teaching which can help us to do this, using the beloved as a mirror. Many of the practices are about learning to totally give or totally receive, to

---

[125] http://www.tantra-essence.com/
[126] http://www.thetantricpath.com/
[127] http://www.tantra.uk.com/

see and be seen, to accept adoration, to acknowledge our beauty. They are also about forgiveness of hurts imposed by either masculine or feminine interactions in our lives (current and potentially past lives too).

There are many tantric exercises about playing within the masculine and feminine roles, and one of the huge gifts that George and I gave each other was that I was a masculine woman whereas he was a feminine man, so to become more masculine than me he had to step far into his masculine character, outside his comfort zone, whereas to become more feminine than him I had to step far into my feminine aspect, way outside my comfort zone. In particular, he showed me it is OK to be vulnerable and to cry. When he did this I loved him all the more. I learned that being vulnerable does not equate to being unlovable, a limiting belief I had carried for many years, and possibly many lifetimes.

With hindsight, what I totally recognise is that I would have not been ready for George if I had met him several years earlier. I had to have done the sexual exploration and initial expansion with Sean, then the work in my psychosynthesis course, and the acceptance of my 'soul' through the out of body and shamanic trainings, before I was ready to jump to the level of sexual awareness and openness and unconditional love and connection with Oneness that George offered. He truly adored me as the embodiment of the feminine. However, he is younger than me and always told me that no matter how much he loved me, he would leave me for a woman who could be the mother of his children, a role I was past fulfilling. Whilst we were together however, I was able to truly let him see me and he was strong enough to act as a mirror to let me see my own shit without judging me or rejecting me for it. What a gift!

This time around, when our relationship ended, I was distraught and my heart was broken again, but I had a much stronger sense of self to support me. An entry from my journal in September 2010, about six weeks after we split up, read, '*I keep bursting into tears. Somehow I need to go into this darkness then find my way out again. I know that help cannot come from outside. I cannot be rescued. Peace, joy, love, acceptance, need to come from within.*'

Of course it is different to know something with the mind and to feel it and live it from the heart, but I did spend the next few months when I was travelling in India, Thailand and Laos, sending George love and wishing for him to be able to fulfil his destiny, have his wife and family, knowing that if he did not truly want to be with me, then I could not be happy with him. How can we ever hold onto someone we profess to love by putting them in a cage? Yet so many people do. That is not love, that is self pity and neediness.

As I write this in 2012 George and I are still extraordinarily close friends. We still have unconditional love for each other and are always there for each other if either one of us asks for any help. There are no strings attached. We recognise that we have been in various relationships with each other over many previous lifetimes (mother, son, father, daughter, friend, lover, victim, perpetrator, murderer, rescuer) and we do not appear to have any karmic debt outstanding. As I wrote in my journal on September 20th, 2010, shortly after I went to India, leaving him in London, *'Over-riding is the sense of our love/connection being much bigger than this lifetime – it seems very old and enduring. He is the embodiment of the masculine to me – at times he seemed to take on the roles of father/son/lover/husband/brother – the embodiment of Shiva.'*

As he put it once shortly after we met, *'We are just two souls who have cleared any karma between us and are available to each other, to help each other from a place of unconditional love.'* That sort of love and connection and communication are, as far as I am aware, extremely rare. I give my thanks.

One of the most basic tantric exercises illustrates well the depth to which our society has sunk regarding the denigration of sex from a joyous, beautiful, sacred act to something dirty and disgusting. In this exercise, the man invites his beloved to lie naked on the bed, in any position he desires, with her legs apart, whilst he admires her body including her feminine organs. No touching. Just looking. Admiring. Honouring. It can of course also be done the other way around, with the woman admiring her partner's genitalia and body.

I suggest this exercise to a number of my clients. Clients who are in relationships or maybe even long term marriages. Almost uniformly a look of horror crosses their faces. They cannot conceive of allowing this! So they allow penetration, intercourse, often very physical abuse of their sexual organs, but they cannot allow the beloved to admire! They usually then admit that they think of their own sexuality as smelly, disgusting, dirty, shameful. Why would their partner want to honour and admire them?

Something has gone horribly wrong.

To heal, to reach our magnificence and our potential, and to love ourselves first so that we may then reach out and love others, we need amongst other things to reach acceptance and love of our physical bodies and our sexual energy, using the latter for love and healing, not for violence and perversion. Tantra to me is about this acceptance. We need to allow ourselves to be truly seen, without shame, without hiding any of our shadow aspects. This has become very difficult for most of us. It is about revealing our true selves, authentically and without fear of judgement. It is about communicating our desires clearly – which of course first requires us to know what our desires truly are. It is about circulating energy between two people to merge their energy fields – a much more profound and erotic connection that the 'friction based' sex we are used to seeing and participating in throughout the Western world.

At the more advanced stages, tantric yoga moves from the individual and the couple to become truly transpersonal, connecting with the quantum universe to reach out to heal all beings in the past, present and future. The metaphor is of Shiva, the divine Father, making love to Shakti, the divine Mother, to create the cosmic universe from which all springs. As with shamanism, in the more advanced exercises we step into being co-creators of our reality, our destiny, and healers of all those connected in the cosmic consciousness.

For instance, during tantric exercises I have worked with forgiveness of all the things that men have done to me as a woman over all my human lifetimes, and then forgiveness of all things all men have done to all women at any time in history. By extension this includes forgiveness of myself and the hurt I have caused to women whilst in a man's body during past lives, thus working for healing in both the present life, the genetic and the karmic lineages.

Whenever this exercise is done, it is done in both directions, so then the men in the group express all the hurt that women have caused them, personally, now and in the past, and then speaking on behalf of all men, at all times. They move on to forgiveness of the feminine, and once again, by extension, forgiveness of themselves in past feminine lives.

This sends out ripples of forgiveness and healing through the universal energy field and for me is a perfect example of the non-sexually based healing intention of tantra. Once again Osho talks of the way love moves from self love, to love of the beloved, to love of the cosmos. *'Falling in love you remain a child; rising in love you mature. And, by and by, love becomes not a relationship, it becomes a state of your being. Then it is not that you love this and you don't love that, no – you are simply love. Whosoever comes near you, you share with them. Whatsoever is happening, you give your love to it. You touch a rock, and you touch as if you are touching your beloved's body. You look at the tree, and you look as if you are looking at your beloved's face. It becomes a state of being. Not that you are 'in love' – now you are love. This is rising; this is not falling.'*[128]

Healing wounded lineages

The healing practices of tantric yoga, shamanism and transpersonal psychotherapy, such as psychosynthesis and family constellations, all believe that once we tap into the all-encompassing energy field, we can heal not only ourselves, but our karmic and genetic lineages.

I described earlier the lineage work I felt I did when using the plant medicine. I am also currently training in constellations therapy, a field pioneered by Bert Hellinger. It looks at the problem facing a client in the wider context of the lineage and its dark secrets, the skeletons in the cupboard which cannot be discussed, the family members who have been ostracised and

---

[128] Osho. 2000. *New Man for the New Millennium.* p.113, Osho International Foundation

excluded. Representatives for the client and for all necessary members of the lineage, or perhaps people they have wronged, are asked to step into what Hellinger labels the 'Knowing Field'. Thousands of case studies have concluded that this work appears to heal all those 'energetically represented' in the constellation, not only the client and the current generation, but the past and future lineages, once again working through space and time.

I first did my own lineage work within the constellation setting with seven generations of women behind me and my daughter in front of me. This particular exercise, which took place as a part of my psychosynthesis training, was one of the most moving single procedures I have ever done. It was also a very profound experience for the other women who were standing in as 'representatives' within my family line. All except one felt it had helped to heal their own feminine lineages, in a perfect example of how this work ripples out beyond the immediate person doing it as a 'client'. During my training I have also experienced the power of the process when standing in as a representative in other people's constellations. It is amazing the information that comes in through the 'Knowing Field' to representatives who are standing in the place of people they intellectually know nothing about and have never met.

Constellations therapist John Payne describes this work as bridging the gap between psychotherapy and shamanism, as the dead are given a voice in the constellation.[129] I totally concur and it has close parallels with one of the shamanic exercises that I do in workshops and with clients, called 'working with the ancestors'. In that exercise, the clients step in to represent their own dead ancestors, but once again they receive information that they were previously unaware of, often from ancestors whom they never met. 'How' is unclear, but the experimental and experiential data base from this work over the last thirty plus years is now huge.[130]

---

[129] Payne, John L. 2005. *The healing of individuals, families and nations*. Forres, Scotland: Findhorn Press

[130] For just one book citing many references, see Franke, Ursula 2003. *The River Never Looks Back. Historical and Practical Foundations of Bert Hellinger's Family Constellations.* Heidelberg, Germany: Carl-Auer-Systeme Verlag

I have also done many past life regressions, some whilst studying Roger Woolger's Deep Memory Process techniques[131]. His way of working calls in victims, perpetrators and family members from many lives, with the healing impact again going well beyond the 'client'.

From dozens of sessions I have observed and participated in, as well as my work with my own clients, I truly believe that many of us at this time are consciously stepping into the role of not only healing ourselves, doing our own work, but also healing our lineages and reaching out to all humanity. I personally know hundreds of people taking on this huge responsibility, through shamanism, tantric yoga, constellations, rebirthing and distance healing. And each of those people probably knows a few hundred more. It is a huge responsibility, but also a huge opportunity, with ripples that travel out non-locally, independent of space and time.

Within the psychosynthesis tradition Piero Ferrucci wrote, *'If you work on yourself, you are already participating in the extraordinary, ageless work of overcoming darkness and pain, and of the evocation of latent potential. Take some time to realize that this work is not only your own private project, but the part of a wider unfoldment in which countless individuals are participating in many ways: the evolution of humankind.'*[132]

There are many ways of working on yourself, and many paths of service to humanity, but tantra seems to me to be one of the most proven and heart-centred ways of recognising the magnificence and potential in ourselves and in all others. In particular, I unreservedly recommend private tantric sessions to any man or woman who has suffered from any sort of sexual abuse or trauma. The level of healing is, in my own personal experience, profound and essential if we are going to love and accept our physical bodies and our sexuality – necessary steps on the journey to truly loving our selves.

I would like to finish this chapter with a quote from Sri Aurobindo, one of the greatest Indian philosophers of recent

---

[131] http://www.deepmemoryprocess.com/

[132] Ferrucci, Piero. 1982. *What we may be.* pp227-228 New York, NY, USA: Jeremy P. Tarcher/Penguin

times, which emphasises the importance of every minute of our lives.

'The soul is not the result of our heredity, but has prepared by its own action and affinities this heredity. It has drawn around it these environmental forces by past karma and consequence. It has created in other lives the mental nature of which now it makes use... To live in this knowledge is not to take away the value and potency of the moment's will and act, but to give it an immensely increased meaning and importance. Then each moment becomes full of things infinite and can be seen taking up the work of a past eternity and shaping the work of a future eternity. Our every thought, will, action carries with it its power of future self-determination and is also a help or a hindrance for the spiritual evolution of those around us and a force in the universal working... Our individual life becomes an immensely greater thing in itself and is convinced too of an abiding unity with the march of the universe.'[133]

[133] Sri Aurobindo. 1952. *The Problem of Rebirth*. pp98-99 Pondicherry, India: Sri Aurobindo Ashram Publication Department

Chapter 14:

Pulling Together the Connections between Altered States of Consciousness, Oneness, the Holographic Universe, Love and Integral Medicine

'Gnosis is knowing we don't know. As we progressively free ourselves from the conceptual matrix we have mistaken for reality, we become certain about less and less until we find ourselves living in the Mystery. It is an extraordinary twist that the great Gnostic injunction 'Know yourself' most famously finds its fulfilment in Socrates, whom the Oracle of Delphi declares the wisest man alive, because 'He knows that he knows nothing'. Gnosis is knowing nothing and loving everything.'[134] (Timothy Freke and Peter Gandy)

'A human being is a part of the whole, called by us the 'universe', a part limited in time and space. He experiences himself, his thoughts and feelings as something separate from the rest – a kind of optical illusion of his consciousness. This delusion is a kind of prison for us, restricting us to our personal

---

[134] Freke, Timothy and Gandy, Peter 2002 *Jesus and the Goddess, The Secret Teachings of the Original Christians.* p.271 London, UK: Thorsons

desires and to affection for a few persons nearest to us. Our task must be to free ourselves from the prison by widening our circle of compassion to embrace all living creatures and the whole of nature in its beauty.[135] (Albert Einstein)

'*A scientific worldview which does not profoundly come to terms with the problem of conscious minds can have no serious pretensions of completeness. Consciousness is part of our universe, so any physical theory which makes a proper place for it falls fundamentally short of providing a genuine description of the world.*'[136] (Sir Roger Penrose)

Once I had been forced by the experiences described in the earlier chapters to accept that I am more than my physical body, the obvious question was, what is it that journeys out of the body and allows me to connect with and collect information from the knowing field, the matrix, the universal energy? What is it that continues from lifetime to lifetime, or, taking a non-linear view of time, is accessible at all times?

We have reached a time when the ancient philosophies and healing methods of the mystics, healers and shamans from many different indigenous peoples are being re-invented by physicists, biologists and psychotherapists. Each group uses different labels and they present their work in different ways, using their own cultural paradigms, but they increasingly acknowledge that there is 'something' universal and eternal that each human being can access if we choose to.

Usually in the meta-physical or religious traditions this 'something' is seen as the omnipresent and omniscient energy that has traditionally been called God, the Creator, the Source, the Divine, the One or Brahman. Many physicists on the other hand label this universal and eternal phenomena the implicate

---

[135] Einstein, Albert. 1972. *New York Post,* November 28
[136] Penrose, Sir Roger *Shadows of the Mind,* quoted in Church Ph.D., Dawson. 2007. *The Genie in Your Genes, Epigenetic Medicine and the New Biology of Intention.* p.161 Llandeilo, U.K.: Cygnus Books

universe, the term coined by Dr. David Bohm. Biologists such as Dr. Candace Pert have named the universal phenomenon the inforealm. Remote viewers such as David Morehouse have named the universal phenomenon the Matrix. Psychotherapists such as Dr. Bert Hellinger call it the Knowing Field. Shamans and energy healers may call it the universal energy or Spirit. All are different labels from very different belief systems, cultures and paradigms, but all seem to be attempting to explain the same phenomenon.

I have come to believe that all of us working and writing in the fields of consciousness, complementary therapy, physics and biology, must be incredibly careful in our use of language with clear definitions when we use words like mind, consciousness, energy, self, information. Many of us think we know what we mean when we use these terms. Unfortunately, we probably mean different things from each other, depending upon which area of specialisation we come from.

This is partly because of ignorance in each area regarding the research that is taking place in the other areas. So for example healers tend to use the word 'energy' when talking about the force that exists non-locally, when 'consciousness' or 'information' might be a more appropriate and less confusing label for those coming from a scientific or medical background. Newer terms such as the 'inforealm' or the 'knowing field' have not yet penetrated the media and public awareness sufficiently widely to be used without significant explanation – although the precision required by explanation might well be helpful in reducing semantic confusion.

Hopefully as we move forward and if I have understood things correctly, the word 'energy' will be more explicitly linked to wave functions within the electro-magnetic spectrum, whilst the labels 'consciousness' and 'information' will spread out from their existing scientific paradigms, to be clearly defined and widely understood within the general public domain.

The Perennial Philosophy and consciousness

Back in 1945 Aldous Huxley coined the term *The Perennial*

Philosophy in his book of that title which was a comparative study of mysticism.[137] He used the term to describe the four fundamental factors he perceived are present in all the major wisdom traditions and religions of the world:

- Consciousness is the fundamental building block of the universe and individualised consciousness is the manifestation of a Divine within which all partial realities exist and apart from which they would be non-existent.
- Human beings are capable of realising the existence of the Divine through their own consciousness, by a direct intuition, superior to reasoning. This immediate knowledge unites the knower with that which is known.
- Humans possess a dual nature, a temporary ego and an eternal self, which is the spark of divinity within the soul.
- Man's life on earth has only one purpose: to identify with his eternal self and so to come to unite with the Divine.

As the evidence of non-locality and Era III healings grows, quantum physics and integral medicine seem to be merging with this perennial mystical philosophy and the religious terms for the universal energy, such as God and the Divine, are increasingly being replaced with the Huxley term, 'consciousness'.

Some of the most famous physicists of the 20th century had already started to openly embrace the quest to connect science, energy fields, consciousness and spirituality. One such example is Erwin Schrodinger, Nobel Laureate physicist, who explained that his discovery of quantum mechanics was an attempt to give form to the central notions of the nondualist, metaphysical philosophy of Advaita, laid forth in the Upanishads.

This Hindu philosophy is based on the fundamental assumption that ultimately all things are one, that the innermost essence of the human being is the very same essence that underlies the universe at large. Within Hinduism that ultimate unity is called Brahman when viewed objectively and Atman when viewed subjectively as the self. Self-realisation brings an

---

[137] Huxley, Aldous. 1945. *The Perennial Philosophy*. USA: Harper and Row

end to suffering and duality. The self is complete in itself, immortal and blissful.

Schrodinger says, '*the reason why our sentient, percipient and thinking ego is met nowhere within our scientific world picture can easily be indicated in seven words: because it is itself that world picture. It is identical with the whole and therefore cannot be contained in it as a part of it. But, of course, here we knock against the arithmetical paradox; there appears to be a great multitude of these conscious egos, the world however is only one.*'[138]

He continues by referring to *The Perennial Philosophy*. '*Open it where you will and you find many beautiful utterances of a similar kind. You are struck by the miraculous agreement between humans of different race, different religion, knowing nothing about each other's existence, separated by centuries and millennia, and by the greatest distances that there are on our globe.*

'*Still, it must be said that to Western thought this doctrine has little appeal, it is unpalatable, it is dubbed fantastic, unscientific. Well, so it is because our science – Greek science – is based on objectivation, whereby it has cut itself off from an adequate understanding of the Subject of Cognizance, of the mind. But I do believe that this is precisely the point where our present way of thinking does need to be amended.*'[139]

In his introduction to *Wholeness and the Implicate Order*, Bohm says, '*I would say that in my scientific and philosophical work, my main concern has been with understanding the nature of reality in general and of consciousness in particular as a coherent whole, which is never static or complete, but which is in an unending process of movement and unfoldment.*'[140]

He examines how consciousness may be understood in relation to the implicate order laid out previously in Chapter 3.

---

[138] Schrodinger, Erwin. 1967. *What is Life? With Mind and Matter and Autobiographical Sketches*. p.128.Cambridge, UK: Cambridge University Press

[139] Schrodinger, Erwin. 1967. *What is Life? With Mind and Matter and Autobiographical Sketches*. pp129-130Cambridge, UK: Cambridge University Press

[140] Bohm, David. 1980. *Wholeness and the Implicate Order*. Introduction p.x U.K: Routledge & Kegan Paul

In this higher dimensional implicate order there are no boundaries of space or time and it appears as if the mind, the body and consciousness are inseparable and ultimately one continuous thing.

The Monroe Institute that I have talked about at length earlier is one important institution that is attempting to bring the different specialisms together to reach a common understanding, collaboratively using the information from all. Another important institution in this field is The Institute of Noetic Sciences[141], founded in 1973 by the Apollo 14 astronaut, Edgar Mitchell. It seeks to further the explorations of conventional science through rigorous enquiry into aspects of reality: mind, consciousness, spirit: that include, yet potentially transcend, physical phenomena.

The book *Consciousness and Healing – Integral Approaches to Mind-Body Medicine,* which I have quoted from a number of times already, is the result of more than three decades of research on consciousness and Era III healing at the Institute.[142]

Elliott Dacher opens the compilation by setting forth four elements that he believes will characterise a post-modern integral medicine: an expanded consciousness, holism, intentionality and a larger self.

He writes, *'An expansion in consciousness is the foundation of a post-modern integral medicine... Through the exploration and full development of consciousness we will at first rediscover the profound and denied inner aspects of healing – wholeness, peace, love, joy and wisdom – and then seamlessly interweave the two traditional aspects of healing – outer and inner – into a new medicine.*

'The modern worldview assumes that outer reality is pre-given, objectified, impersonal, measurable, quantifiable, and ultimately knowable through our sensory perceptions. The post-modern view does not make this assumption. Objective and subjective, outer and inner, are seen as inseparable and seamless

---

[141] www.noetic.org
[142] Schlitz, Marilyn and Amorok, Tina with Micozzi, Marc S. 2005. *Consciousness and Healing.* St Louis, Missouri, USA: Elsevier

experiences, with each shaping the other in an ongoing circularity of movement...

'The modern worldview postulates that all phenomena are caused by unchanging universal laws that exist independently of human consciousness... The post-modern perspective validates and legitimizes the causal nature of consciousness that is individually willed and downward in direction. In validating both downward and upward causation we affirm and expand our understanding of the mind-body unity and simultaneously affirm and expand our capacity for self-regulation.'[143]

As I understand his writing, Dossey too appears to have come to the conclusion that consciousness is the best term for the non-local awareness mechanism which underpins Era III healings. He reviews twelve scientists' models of consciousness that embody this non-local quality of the mind. I paraphrase a selection of them from his book below, but they all agree that consciousness is fundamental and unconstrained by space or time:[144]

- David J. Chalmers, a mathematician and cognitive scientist from the University of Arizona, suggested that consciousness is fundamental in the universe and is not derived from anything else, and cannot be reduced to anything more basic, freeing it from its local confinement to the brain.[145]
- Nobel physicist Brian D Josephson of Cambridge University's Cavendish Laboratory has proposed that non-local events not only exist at the subatomic level but, through the actions of the mind, can be amplified and emerge in our everyday experience as distant mental events of a broad variety.[146]

---

[143] Schlitz, Marilyn and Amorok, Tina with Micozzi, Marc S.. 2005. *Consciousness and Healing.* pp10-11 St Louis, Missouri, USA: Elsevier

[144] Dossey, Dr., Larry. 2009. *Healing Beyond the Body.* pp211-213 London, UK: Piatkus Books

[145] Chalmers, David J. 1995. The Puzzle of Conscious Experience. *Scientific American* 273, no 6: pp80-86

[146] Josephson, Brian D. and Pallikara-Viras, F. 1991. Biological Utilization of Quantum Nonlocality. *Foundations of Physics* 21. pp197-207

- Systems theorist Ervin Lazlo has proposed that non-local, consciousness-mediated events such as intercessory prayer, telepathy, precognition and clairvoyance may be explainable through developments in physics concerning the quantum vacuum and zero-point field.[147]
- Robert G Jahn and his colleagues at the Princeton Engineering Anomalies Research lab have proposed a model of the mind in which consciousness acts freely through space and time to create actual change in the physical world. Their hypothesis is based on their experimental evidence, which is the largest database ever assembled of the effects of distant intentionality.[148]
- Sir James Jeans, the British mathematician, astronomer and physicist, says in *Physics and Philosophy* that when we view ourselves in space and time, our consciousnesses are the separate individuals of a particle picture, but when we pass beyond space and time, they may perhaps form ingredients of a single continuous stream of life. As it is with light and electricity, so it may be with life: the phenomena may be individuals carrying on separate existences in space and time, while in the deeper reality beyond space and time we may all be members of one body.[149]

Physiology and consciousness

So, if consciousness is omnipresent and omniscient, how does that fit in with the physiology of the brain and what we often refer to as mind?

Within the brain each cell has a skeletal structure and the

---

[147] Lazlo, Ervin. 1995. *Interconnected Universe: Conceptual Foundations of Transdisciplinary Unified Theory.* N.J. USA: River Edge World Scientific
[148] Jahn, Robert G. and. Dunne, Brenda J 1987. *Margins of Reality: The Role of Consciousness in the Physical World.* New York, N.Y., USA: Harcourt Brace Jovanovich
[149] Sir Jeans, James. 1981. *Physics and Philosophy.* New York, N.Y., USA: Dover

shape of the cell is partially determined by a system of rigid, cylindrical protein beams called microtubules. Recent research has confirmed that microtubules are transient and are frequently rebuilt, in some cells several times an hour.

Writing about the microtubules of the brain in the *Science and Consciousness Review*, John McCrone questions the implications of the fact that the average half-life of these microtubules is just ten minutes between assembly and destruction.

'*Now the brain is supposed to be some sort of computer. It is an intricate network of some 1000 trillion synaptic connections, each of these synapses having been lovingly crafted by experience to have a particular shape, a particular neurochemistry. It is of course the information represented at these junctions that makes us who we are. But how the heck do these synapses retain a stable identity when the chemistry of cells is almost on the boil, with large molecules falling apart nearly as soon as they are made?*

'*The issue of molecular turnover is starting to hit home in neuroscience, especially now that the latest research techniques such as fluorescent tagging are revealing a far more frantic pace of activity than ever suspected. For instance the actin filaments in dendrites can need replacing within 40 seconds... (and) ... the entire post-synaptic density (PSD), the protein packed zone that powers synaptic activity, is replaced, molecule for molecule, almost by the hour*'.[150]

With the entire brain being reconstructed about once a month, how does our neurological mind retain its knowledge and memory?

As I understand it, Pert believes it is because the neurological mind is simply the machine that connects with the external hard drive where the information is stored – what I have been referring to as consciousness, but which she labels the inforealm. '*The mind as we experience it is immaterial, yet it has a physical substrate, which is both the body and the brain. It may also be said to have a nonmaterial, nonphysical substrate that has to do with the flow of that information. The mind, then, is that which holds the network together, often acting below our consciousness,*

---

[150] McCrone, John. 2004. How do you persist when your molecules don't? *Science and Consciousness Review*. www.sci-con.org/articles/20040601.html

linking and coordinating the major systems and their organs and cells in an intelligently orchestrated symphony of life. Thus we might refer to the whole system as a psychosomatic information network, linking psyche, which comprises all that is of an ostensibly nonmaterial nature, such as mind, emotion and soul, to soma, which is the material world of molecules, cells and organs.'[151]

At a later date, with Henry Dreher and Michael Ruff, Pert writes, *'The word 'soul' is still assiduously avoided by academic scientists. But what animates the neuropeptides in their flow patterns through the body? What animates the receptors? These flexible cell-surface molecules vibrate, shimmy, and even hum as they change shapes, awaiting arrival of their matching ligands. The entire healing system is propelled by chemical energies, but to reverse the usual question: What is the immaterial substrate of these ceaseless biochemical reactions?'*[152]

They believe the answer lies in an information-based paradigm with information being the unifying concept that spans the emotional, energetic, biochemical, molecular and genetic levels of the human system.

Church quotes further evidence about the interaction of microtubules and the life-force energy field, collected by Robin Kelly, a British physician. *'Kelly describes how 'in the early 1990s a British physicist, Sir Roger Penrose, joined forces with an American anaesthetist, Dr. Stuart Hameroff, as both were intrigued by these microtubules... They 'developed the hypothesis that these hollow tubes were our body's link with consciousness – an environment where the timeless quantum world was allowed to collapse down to our recognizable physical world of time and space.'*[153] *While the resonant properties of microtubules is a subject still awaiting serious research scrutiny, it is possible*

---

[151] Pert Ph.D., Candace B. 1999. *Molecules of Emotion, Why You Feel the Way You Feel.* p185 London, U.K.: Simon & Schuster

[152] Pert, Candace B., Dreher, Henry E. and Ruff, Michael R. 2005. The Psychosomatic Network: Foundations of Mind-Body Medicine. pp77-78 in *Consciousness and Healing*, edited by Schlitz, Marilyn and Amorok, Tina with Micozzi, Marc S. St Louis, Missouri, USA: Elsevier

[153] Kelly, Robin. 2006. *The Human Aerial.* p.89 New Zealand: Zenith

that they may play a role in the transmission of intention and consciousness across distances.' [154]

As with non-locality and Era III healings, the questions about how our brains and our bodies retain memory when they are constantly in a state of flux and reconstruction seem obvious, the answers much less so! Hopefully this will be an area where the research doctors and scientists can come forth with an explanation in terminology that the general public can understand. Meantime, as a non-doctor, the fact that the inforealm is situated outside the physical body seems to me to give hope to those incapacitated by memory loss – although connection with that inforealm would potentially be enhanced through research on the impact of some of the natural plants that are currently classified as too dangerous to use!

[154] Church Ph.D., Dawson. 2007. *The Genie in Your Genes, Epigenetic Medicine and the New Biology of Intention.* p.194 Llandeilo, U.K.: Cygnus Books

Chapter 15:
My New Life as a Shaman

'*Our deepest fear is not that we are inadequate. Our deepest fear is that we are powerful beyond measure. It is our light, not our darkness that most frightens us. We ask ourselves, 'Who am I to be brilliant, gorgeous, talented, fabulous?' Actually, who are you not to be? ... Your playing small does not serve the world.*'[155] (Marianne Williamson)

The more I read and learn and explore, the more I recognise that all the ancient wisdoms teach the same basics, as expounded by Huxley in *The Perennial Philosophy*. They accept that:

- we are more than our physical bodies
- we are part of one consciousness that moves throughout the cosmos (whether or not that consciousness can be described as energy being open to discussion as quantum physics evolves)
- we carry pain and suffering from life to life, repeating patterns over and over again until we are ready to look at them, acknowledge them, integrate their gifts and lessons and let go of their negative aspects, aspects that may have served us in the past, but no longer do so
- we are here to evolve and grow, to become aware, to live

---

[155] Williamson, Marianne. 1996. *A Return to Love.* pp190-19 USA: Harper Collins

our lives consciously, for ourselves and all others. Indeed eventually to realise there are no others, to reach a place of Unity rather than Duality.

In *The Call*, Oriah Mountain Dreamer asks each one of us to remember the one word we are here to say with our whole being.[156] To find your word she recommends looking at your failures, at the places where you most easily go to sleep and become unconscious about what you are doing. What does not come easily to you, what do you long for but find elusive, what gets you into trouble, what gets you way down the road of doing something you don't really want to do at a very high price? What repeatedly robs your life of joy?

Reading *The Call* a few years ago I knew almost straight away what my word was. It was surrender. For many years I had fought to control, to organise, to be accepted, to be right. What I need to live is surrender.

We are in control of very little and our attempts to control others, let alone the wider world, merely cause antagonism, pain and rejection when others find our efforts to impose **our** way unacceptable.

Plans written in stone rob our lives of spontaneity, force us into doing what was decided beforehand rather than what the moment requires.

Doing what we think we need to do to be accepted by others is handing over our power, our responsibility, our lives. Those who choose to judge our actions without understanding them are imposing their belief system on us and saying only their way is right. And of course when we say we are right, we are implying others are wrong. But right and wrong are highly subjective, words and concepts coloured by our culture, our personal experiences and perspectives.

Surrender for me is difficult to implement. It means I need to live each moment as if it may be my last in this lifetime. I need to make each moment count, finding the joy, the beauty, the peace,

---

[156] Mountain Dreamer, Oriah. 2010. *The Call – Discovering Why You Are Here*. USA: Harper Collins

the pleasure, the lesson in what is **right now**. Contrary to my old life in the corporate world, living in surrender is what I now try to do each day of my life, supported by my shamanic practices.

This does not mean I hand over responsibility to the Divine (let alone any other human being), sit back and let someone else take care of me. It means working with whatever hand I get dealt at any time, working with what is, not what I would like it to be, and if something isn't to be, I try not to waste precious moments trying to change it and make it happen. What I do each moment does still have potential consequences in the future, each action increases the probability of certain future outcomes whilst diminishing the probability of others, but I try always to live in the moment, not constantly worrying about what I could have/should have done differently in the past and not thinking constantly about what might or might not emerge in the future. I just need to do the best I can at any moment, with the resources I have available right now.

Personally I recognise that I'm not too bad about letting go of the past, not dwelling in what could have been different. Because shit happens. I try not to get stuck in it or carry it around with me.

However I do acknowledge and recognise that I'm very bad at not dreaming about the future. I still run stories in my head, scenarios. *'When I meet this person again I am going to say or do this and that, then they will say or do this and that, then the evening will end up like this or that and then the outcome for my life will be*...(whatever little story I have made up in my head to suit my own desires)'.

You know what?

Things never work out the way I have spent hours imagining and agonising over. The other person has their own agenda. They never act the way I have dreamt up or say what I have created in my head. It is a total waste of my time and energy, using up a moment that will never come again. Living in the future like this prevents me from living in the now.

Surrender is about experiencing to the full **what is,** not trying to constrain the world to be what we would like it to be.

In *What We May Be*, Piero Ferrucci uses the word acceptance rather than surrender, but it appears to me to represent the same intention. '*When an unpleasant event happens to us, we can decide to accept it as it is, without complaining, because the universe does not adjust itself to our plans... Our first spontaneous reaction may of course be one of self-pity, evasion or rebellion. But as we assume a positive, dynamic attitude of acceptance (not resignation or approval) we find we can better understand what is coming our way, learn from its message, take advantage of the hidden circumstances it may offer, and if we so decide, fight it effectively. In any case we will be able to take responsibility for whatever choice we in fact have – choice about our actions, thoughts and feelings – instead of simply blaming everything on the outside world.*'[157]

'*Acceptance becomes the quickest and most practical way to free oneself from a difficult situation, while rebellion inexorably tightens the knot. The transition from rebellion to acceptance may have an extremely important consequence: the shift from a reactive to a cognitive attitude, in which we see life as a training school, where a series of situations tends to teach us exactly what we need to learn.*

'*Painful situations then become charades to be deciphered rather than nuisances to curse at. And instead of merely surviving by being hurt, weary or frustrated, we can emerge from them enriched and with greater understanding.*'[158]

Surrender to me also means going into my Higher Self, finding out what will feel right for me to do, what will let me live in peace and happiness and then acting on that, without worrying if the world thinks I've gone mad. That is not arrogance, although I can see how it could be perceived as that. For me it's the way to a much calmer, less stressed, more considerate, less judgemental, more connected and authentic way of living.

Another word that has come up many times, with different teachers, is 'joy'. Is this just by chance that so many intuitive people perceive I have issues with joy, or is it because they can tap into my energetic field and sense a deep block?

---

[157] Ferrucci, Piero. 1982. *What we may be.* p.114 New York, NY, USA: Jeremy P. Tarcher/Penguin

[158] Ferrucci, Piero. 1982. *What we may be.* p.115 New York, NY, USA: Jeremy P. Tarcher/Penguin

In 2008 my rebirthing teacher said that when she looked at me she saw a very sad aura, and I came across as very serious, sober, puritanical, with very little joy. I responded that I felt very blessed and happy. But she re-iterated that that was not what I was conveying to the outside observer. It did very much resonate with my old 'story' of all joy being sinful. The phrase I took out of that session was 'lighten up'. Be happier, not so serious all the time.

It also fitted in with the guilt I had felt in the psychosynthesis groups that I attended as part of my training, when I felt my life was beautiful and almost perfect, yet I found it hard to voice this when everyone around was complaining about their problems and their misery. Somehow I still carried a belief that it was not okay to be happy (although it was fine for a 'good girl' to be miserable).

The issue of joylessness recurred in a shamanic training in 2007 where it appeared to emanate from a very ancient wounding and soul contract. The lost soul part at the time of that particular wounding was a very small child full of love and joy and light, who had been ceremoniously mutilated by her tribe. That separated soul part was not sure about coming back to re-integrate into my current life. I work too hard, I am too serious, I don't have a sense of humour, I am no fun. The separated or lost soul part was not sure I would give it space, I was too much focused on results, on doing. I had to promise to lighten up, to bring joy into my life every day and sometimes to do nothing at all, just be.

I so wish that as a child someone had introduced me to the words of shamanic counsellor Kenneth Meadows and one of his Native American teachers, Silver Bear. '*But what is the purpose of it all? Part of the answer was given to me in two simple words: 'To enjoy'. To enjoy? But haven't we been given to believe that life was intended to be a struggle to endure, to control and subjugate? That is a false concept. A purpose of life is to enjoy aliveness. To enjoy pleasure. Not in the sense of self-indulgence, but in the knowledge that joy, excitement and fulfilment from exploring, discovering and creating are what life was given to us for. Self-development comes through experiencing the conditions and circumstances we create for ourselves as a result of our own creativeness. Silver Bear explained. 'You are constantly creating yourself with every moment. You change your Fate, your direction, your circumstances, your environment, by changing your thoughts. Never forget – the power is in the Now. Power always lies in the Present.'* [159]

One last word that I have worked with on many occasions over the last few years is 'vulnerability'. The Corporate Bitch would never have shown vulnerability. That would have implied weakness and she would have assumed it would have given 'others' an opportunity to attack her and bring her down. I lived in a world where I believed I was in constant competition for insufficient resources – be they financial or emotional.

Being vulnerable was the same as being pathetic.

Being vulnerable was the same as being unlovable.

Over the years I have observed and worked with so many people, men and women, who hold these same beliefs.

But actually we all like to be useful and take care of others and only when someone asks us for help are we able to give it. By refusing to be vulnerable or needy, by refusing to receive, we prevent any others from giving. George was the man who initially showed me that being vulnerable is not weak and is certainly not unlovable. We all need help at times and we all have gifts and strength to offer at times. In a world where people recognise their interconnectedness, the ebb and flow of giving and receiving would be a natural part, rather than each individual trying to accumulate as much as possible for themselves, at the expense of others.

My intention in writing this book is to pass on the gifts and teachings I have received to others, particularly those who have never been exposed to the new biologies of psycho-neuroimmunology and epigenetics, quantum physics and altered states of consciousness.

I just pray that my own story and the evidence I have presented will encourage you to read some of the sources I have quoted and from which I have learned, expanding your

---

[159] Meadows, Kenneth. 1990. *The Medicine Way, A Shamanic Path to Self Mastery.* p.114 Shaftsbury, Dorset, U.K.: Element Books Limited

knowledge and opening you to the possibility of exploring your own Higher Self, to continuing your own path of development and growth and to living with love and compassion, with humility and curiosity.

People sometimes ask me if I regret the fact that I now live in a little house rather than a mansion with a swimming pool? Do I miss the fine wining and dining? Am I worried about my financial future which looks relatively precarious?

Absolutely not! I live an almost completely stress free life, doing a job I love, with the honour of hearing people's most intimate stories and helping them to release their pain and their suffering and their limiting beliefs in order to realise their potential. I don't have to get up at 6am and return home exhausted at 7pm. I get up around 8am, go running in the beautiful park very close to my house, come home, have a leisurely breakfast, shower, dress in whatever I feel like wearing for the day (be that jeans or a Goddess dress), take my dog for a walk, then come back and see my clients. I read, play the piano and go dancing. I surround myself socially with like-minded, nurturing friends, who are also on a path of connection and awareness. I buy very little as I really don't need much 'stuff', and I go away to beautiful parts of the world for several months a year to continue my own journey of exploration and learning. Indeed I have now started leading journeys to Peru with my clients, to allow them to enter into ceremony with the Shipibo shamans and their plant medicine, with the Qero and their healing. I feel incredibly blessed and honoured.

Old friends say I seem happier and more peaceful than ever before. I feel I have a purpose and whilst some of my friends are reaching retirement, I am just starting on my new profession which I don't believe will ever end as long as I am in this physical body.

To be of service effectively, I have to live the way of the shaman: live as love, seeing the beauty in every person, every thing, every situation, with gratitude for being allowed to sing the song of life in this body for another day, on this beautiful planet, at this amazing time of transformation.

I also need to surround myself with natural beauty such as flowers, shells, candles, music. I need to live consciously, saying yes to life, recognising that each day is precious as it will never come again, and that what I do each day impacts not only my current life, but my past lives and my future lives too, as well as my ancestors and my lineage. All my words and my thoughts impact those they are directed at and so every word, thought and action needs to be done consciously, with awareness of the potential impact.

Two of my biggest lessons have been to appreciate how little I truly know or control and to honour the miracle of the universal energy field, consciousness or inforealm within which we are tiny, interconnected sparks.

I would like to finish with a final quote from Osho.

'Anything that helps you to attain the fulfilment of your potential is good. It is not only a blessing to you, it is a blessing to the whole existence. No man is an island. We are all a vast infinite continent, joined together in the roots. Maybe our branches are separate, but our roots are one. Realising one's potential is the only morality there is. Losing one's potential and falling into darkness and retardedness is the only sin, the only evil.'[160]

Namaste – from the Goddess in me to the Divine in you.

---

[160] Osho. 2000. *New Man for the New Millennium.* p.183 Osho International Foundation

Glossary

Atman: The Higher Self, the Permanent Self, which survives after physical death. The Atman can travel through space and time, can be launched from one dimension of existence into another and can take up residence time after time in different human bodies to experience the realm of matter and thereby further its development or evolution.

Attunement: The Reiki term for being opened to receiving and using Reiki energy for healing. The level 1 attunement allows self healing, the level 2 attunement allows healing of others and the level 3 attunement allows you to pass on the Reiki teachings and attune others.

Ayahuasca: A hallucinogenic plant found in the Amazon containing di-methytriptamine. It is used by the shamans for journeying outside the body and communicating with plants and animals and their wisdom.

Ayurveda: The science of life, deriving from the Sanskrit terms 'ayur' meaning life and 'veda' meaning science or knowledge.

Bardo: A resting or waiting place between lives.

Biological or genealogical lineage: Our bloodline ancestors, mother, father, grandparents, great-grandparents and so on.

Brahman: The Hindu term for the innermost essence of all things, the ultimate unity, which manifests in individuals as Atman.

Chakra: Energy centre reaching from within the physical body outwards in a cone shape through the various energy layers that surround the physical body.

Cosmos: All manifest existence.

Epigenetics: The science of how environmental signals select, modify and regulate gene activity leading to heritable changes in gene function that occur without a change in the DNA sequence.

Explicate Order: The normal, large scale, three dimensional world.

Focus level: A term used at the Monroe Institute to label different states of consciousness. At focus fifteen you step outside linear space and time, at focus twenty-one you cross between the living and the dead and at focus twenty-seven you reach the resting place for regeneration between lives and decisions regarding your next incarnation, whether in human or alternate form.

Gnosis: Awareness, consciousness or enlightenment.

Higher Self: See Atman.

Hologram: Three dimensional photos and when you tilt them, or move past them, the image inside appears to move. A permanent record of what something looks like in three dimensions.

Holotropic breathwork: A way of breathing evolved by Stanislav Grof as a way of accessing altered states of consciousness.

Implicate Order: David Bohm coined the term implicate order to describe a model of the universe where each region contains a total structure enfolded within it.

Karma: The totality of our actions and their accompanying reactions in this, previous and future lives.

Karmic Lineage: The succession of past lives a person has lived.

Kundalini: A Sanskrit word meaning coiled up, like a snake or a spring. It is traditionally symbolised as a sleeping serpent coiled at the base of the human spine, with the potential to rise through the chakras to the crown allowing the bio-energy to rise and assist on the path to transformation and enlightenment.

Metaphysics: A branch of philosophy dealing with the cause and nature of being, what is reality?

Nadi: The system of energy channels superimposed on the physical body.

Non-locality: A measurement at one point in space can influence what occurs at another point in space even if the distance between the points is large enough so that no signal can travel between them at light speed in the time allowed for measurement.

Paradigm: A pattern, model, exemplar.

Psychoneuroimmunology (PNI): The medical research which connects our thoughts (psyche), our nervous system (neurology) and our immune system.

Psychosynthesis: The realisation of individual and collective potential and the harmonisation of all elements of the personality.

Quantum entanglement: The interconnectedness of all particles in the universe.

Quantum physics: The branch of physics involving the study of the subatomic realm.

Reiki: Literally translated, universal life force. It is a method of energy healing at the physical, mental and emotional level and can be conducted remotely as well as in the same room as the client. It is activated by intention and presence.

Shaman: A healer capable of working outside space and time.

Synchronicity: A coincidence that has a personal meaning beyond the immediate facts of the situation.

Tantra: Liberation through expansion. A spiritual path for attaining enlightenment or union with the divine.

Transpersonal: Beyond the personal, connecting with all of humanity and the cosmos.

Upanishads: The holy books of India, the basis of Hinduism, deriving from several thousand years B.C.

Bibliography

Begg, Deike. 1999. *Rebirthing, Freedom From Your Past*. London, UK: Thorsons

Begg, Deike. 2004. *Synchronicity: The Promise of Coincidence*. UK: Chiron Publications

Bohm, David. 1980. *Wholeness and the Implicate Order*. UK: Routledge & Kegan Paul

Brennan, Barbara Ann. 1988. *Hands of Light*. USA and Canada: Bantam Books

Buchanan, Lyn. 2003. *The Seventh Sense, The Secrets of Remote Viewing as Told by a 'Psychic Spy' for the U.S. Military*. New York, NY, USA: Paraview Pocket Books

Church, Dawson. 2007. *The Genie in Your Genes, Epigenetic Medicine and the New Biology of Intention*. Llandeilo, UK: Cygnus Books

Dossey, Dr., Larry. 2009. *Healing Beyond the Body*. London, UK: Piatkus Books

Dossey, Dr., Larry. 1997. *Prayer is Good Medicine*. New York, NY, USA: Harper Collins

Ferrucci, Piero. 1982. *What we may be*. New York, NY, USA: Jeremy P. Tarcher/Penguin

Franke, Ursula. 2003. *The River Never Looks Back. Historical and Practical Foundations of Bert Hellinger's Family Constellations*. Heidelberg, Germany: Carl-Auer-Systeme Verlag

Freke, Timothy and Gandy, Peter. 2002. *Jesus and the Goddess, The Secret Teachings of the Original Christians*. London, UK: Thorsons

Hawking, Stephen and Mlodinow, Leonard. 2010. *The Grand Design*. London, UK: Bantam Press

Huxley, Aldous. 1945. *The Perennial Philosophy*. USA: Harper and Row

Jahn, Robert G. and. Dunne, Brenda J. 1987. *Margins of Reality: The Role of Consciousness in the Physical World.* New York, NY, USA: Harcourt Brace Jovanovich

Sir Jeans, James. 1981. *Physics and Philosophy.* New York, NY, USA: Dover

Kelly, Robin. 2006. *The Human Aerial.* New Zealand: Zenith

Lazlo, Ervin. 1995. *Interconnected Universe: Conceptual Foundations of Transdisciplinary Unified Theory.* NJ, USA: River Edge World Scientific

Lipton Ph.D., Bruce H. 2005. *The Biology of Belief.* Carlsbad, CA, USA: Hay House, Inc.

McMoneagle, Joseph. 1993. *Mind Trek, Exploring Consciousness, Time and Space Through Remote Viewing.* Charlottesville, VA, USA: Hampton Roads

Meadows, Kenneth. 1990. *The Medicine Way, A Shamanic Path to Self Mastery.* Shaftsbury, Dorset, UK: Element Books Limited

Monroe, Robert A. 1971. *Journeys out of the Body.* USA: Doubleday

Monroe, Robert A. 1985. *Far Journeys.* USA: Doubleday

Monroe, Robert A. 1994. *Ultimate Journey.* USA: Doubleday

Morehouse, David. 2000. *Psychic Warrior, the true story of the CIA's paranormal espionage programme.* UK: Clairview

Mountain Dreamer, Oriah. 2010. *The Call – Discovering Why You Are Here.* USA: Harper Collins

Narby, Jeremy. 1999. *The Cosmic Serpent, DNA and the Origins of Knowledge.* New York, NY, USA: Jeremy P. Tarcher/Putnam

Osho. 1973. *From Sex to Superconsciousness.* Pune, MS, India: Osho Media International

Osho. 1974. *The Book of Secrets.* New York NY, USA: Osho International Foundation

Osho. 2000. *New Man for the New Millennium.* Penguin Books

Payne, John L. 2005. *The healing of individuals, families and nations.* Forres, Scotland: Findhorn Press

Pert Ph.D., Candace B. 1999. *Molecules of Emotion, Why You Feel the Way You Feel.* London, UK: Simon & Schuster

Schlitz, Marilyn, Amorok, Tina with Micozzi, Marc S. 2005. *Consciousness and Healing.* St Louis, Missouri, USA: Elsevier

Schrodinger, Erwin. 1967. *What is Life? With Mind and Matter and Autobiographical Sketches.* Cambridge, UK: Cambridge University Press

Shealy, M.D., Ph.D., Norman and Church Ph.D., Dawson. 2008. *Soul Medicine: Awakening your Inner Blueprint for Abundant Health and Energy.* USA: Energy Psychology Press

Singh Khalsa, M.D., Dharma and Stauth, Cameron 2001. *Meditation as Medicine.* New York, NY, USA: Fireside

Sri Aurobindo. 1952. *The Problem of Rebirth.* Pondicherry, India: Sri Aurobindo Ashram Publication Department

Strassman, M.D., Rick. 2001. *DMT: The Spirit Molecule – A Doctor's Revolutionary Research into the Biology of Near-Death and Mystical Experiences.* Rochester, Vermont, USA: Park Street Press

Targ, Russell. 2004. *Limitless Mind, a guide to remote viewing and transformation of consciousness.* Novato, CA, USA: New World Library

Williamson, Marianne. 1996. *A Return to Love.* USA: Harper Collins

Villoldo, Ph.D., Alberto. 2005. *Mending the Past and Healing the Future with Soul Retrieval.* Carlsbad, CA, USA: Hay House, Inc

Williamson, Marianne. 1996. *A Return to Love.* USA: Harper Collins

Useful Sources

American Holistic Medical Association
http://www.holisticmedicine.org/content.asp?pl=2&sl=43&con
tentid=43

Ashi Meraya – Amazon plant medicine retreat centre
http://www.elmundomagico.org/ashi-meraya-centre-of-
traditional-amazonian-medicine/

Association for Comprehensive Energy Psychology
http://www.energypsych.org/

**Capacitar – A core program of energy-based healing practices
that awaken and empower people**
http://www.capacitar.org/index.html

Epigenome Network of Excellence
http://www.epigenome.eu

Four Winds Society
http://www.thefourwinds.com/

John Hawken
http://www.thetantricpath.com/

Holos University
http://www.holosuniversity.org/index.php

Institute of Noetic Sciences
http://www.noetic.org

Ma Ananda Sarita
http://www.tantra-essence.com/

Monroe Institute
http://www.monroeinstitute.org/research/overview-of-research-at-the-monroe-institute

Peruvian Munay Ki rites
http://www.munay-ki.org

Soul Medicine Institute
http://www.soulmedicineinstitute.org/

Transcendence: Authentic tantra yoga
http://www.tantra.uk.com/